The
ORIGINS
of
ILLNESS

Fulton Books, Inc.
Meadville, PA

Published by Fulton Books 2020

ISBN 978-1-64654-128-7 (paperback)
ISBN 978-1-64654-129-4 (digital)

Printed in the United States of America

Ranveig Elvebakk, MD

The
ORIGINS
of
ILLNESS

Health and Illness in the Quantum Era

Edited by Doris Mehler

To my husband, Thomas Farren, without whose razor-
sharp sense of logic and insight this book would not be.

CONTENTS

FOREWORD

Even before I became a medical doctor, I was convinced that rather than diagnoses and pictures in a pathology book, illnesses are processes that can be understood and manipulated.

To grasp this, we have to accept some concepts of modern physics not yet acknowledged by medicine. We have to think of ourselves as part of the holistic living ecosystem.

We tend to think of this as "new wave." However, holism finds its explanation in principles of quantum theory that connect us all.

Life is an endless stream of oncoming energies or possibilities that we chose from with wide-reaching and sometimes unpredicted consequences for us and everyone around us. Our fate is intertwined with, and cannot be separated from, that of the planet. The better we understand this connectedness, the wiser our choices.

Simply expressed, our health is a lifelong energy exchange between the body and the environment. The better we manage this exchange, the healthier we will be.

The purpose of this book is to show how we can use this information to bring the energy of healing to all areas of our lives. This information should be available to people of all ages and start in schools as the famous "ounce of prevention".

My own journey to this understanding came through my work in clinical medicine where the reactions of exposing the body to different substances could be measured. In my work with weight and nutrition I saw the power of nutrition to reverse illness.

It all added up to the realization that by understanding the causes of illnesses rather than inventing fixes, we can rid ourselves of the majority of our disease-burden. A library of modern science supports this thinking.

It is my hope that we can leave pride, personality and prejudice behind and use this information to take ownership of our health and that of the planet.

CHAPTER 1
The Doctrines that Limit Us

From time immemorial, human beings have sought to understand the world and the forces that rule it. We struggle to reconcile with nature's apparently inexplicable whims from natural disasters to personal tragedy. Our human mind is not geared toward uncertainty and coincidence; they produce fear. It looks for the predictable and instinctually recognizable. We seek safety through certainty and explanations.

A common philosophical expression of this is determinism. Everything is linearly predetermined and predictable from the past and the present, setting the stage for a future where we might have at best limited influence by virtue of understanding the past. Absent true clarity, we are left lending divine significance to unrelated events to explain the unexplainable. The purest form of determinism is fatalism, often ritualized into religion, whereby we surrender to the will of an all-knowing, all-powerful deity. Things are meant to be and happen for reasons known only to the divine being. This world view transcends all belief and philosophy, especially in times of untimely illness or death, which are still seen as punishment in some settings, including within Christian doctrine.

The Strong Get Stronger

With his discovery of the laws of gravity and motion, Isaac Newton put a new spin on determinism that seemed to corroborate the view that life unfolds in a linear fashion. The ability to assess and measure natural events was confirmation of this order, and it provided definition, even description and numeration. The world became the eternal clockwork set in motion by the divine hand at the beginning of time and ticking toward eternity. The ultimate interpretation of this is that everything began with the big bang and is still unfolding according to plan.

Determinism was again reinforced by Darwin's theory of the evolution of the species and his thesis of natural selection. This became "darwinism." Life is a draconian competition where some have the superior ability to survive and reproduce. It was seized on by philosophers such as Herbert Spencer, and the social dogma of the survival of the fittest was born. The world is divided into the winners who, by virtue of their given attributes adjust faster and more successfully to their environment, especially economically, while the losers fall behind.

The opposing view was expressed some fifty years earlier by the French botanist Jean-Baptiste Lamarck. Foreshadowing epigenetics, Lamarck realized that the environment changes characteristics of living cells without changing the genes, so-called soft inheritance. He pointed out the evolutionary advantages of what he called instructive cooperation among organisms. This implies that we all can learn, contribute to and enhance evolution by cooperation. It not only enables the survival of the species, but shifts the mode from survival to thrive and has helped humankind rise to the top of the food chain. He furthermore pointed out that these changes are passed on to future generations. However, his work fell outside the accepted dogma and was dismissed and forgotten.

We have expounded on the Newtonian and Darwinian foundations. They are offered up as proof that man is selfish, greedy and brutal as a matter of course. They disregard the duality of our nature and our capacity for an entire range of behavior around a given attribute and conclude that our competitive instincts and greed will dominate.

This interpretation is probably singlehandedly the most damaging doctrine in recent human history, creating chasms instead of coherence. It negates the idea that we all can aspire to a higher purpose. We believe that a system of shared wealth is ruinous to our culture.

This belief has become so pervasive and engrained in our psyche that it is part of our collective consciousness.

It is our modus operandi and the philosophical foundation of numerous extreme theories within the political, social and economic realm, including that of racial supremacy. Co-opted in the nineteenth century, it became the moral justification for the social inequities seen then, and has persisted, fueling the so-called Gilded Age. We are currently living the resurgence of this philosophy, though some rethinking seems to be in the offing.

Medicine Joins the Bandwagon

In medicine the determinist evolutionism was corroborated by the discovery of the genome. Unfortunately, our interpretation of genes was the next major calamity in the history of humanity and the development of medicine. In fact, it still is. Genes were touted as the master blueprint for our lives. Even today they are erroneously thought of as masters of our cells, attributed with the power to run our bodies and define our lives. We now have the physical explanation for our destiny. Hence, we assign everything from our health and illness to social status to our genetic makeup. It is confirmation of the fact that some of us are born sickly, cruel or poor with no ability to change it.

Only recently have we come to appreciate that the discovery of the genome was only a crude beginning of our understanding of genetics. It would take half a century before we found out how genes actually work. Yet we fervently cling to our genetic destiny.

The Genius of Genes

In order to understand genes, we have to discuss their distribution and relation to our body. It consists at its core of hundreds of thousands of specialized proteins tasked with different missions ranging from supplying our body structure to messengers and carriers that run it. For this reason, we have been called protein machines. Proteins are strands of amino acids in very specific order.

Much like a computer program, genes are pieces of code, dictating the order of amino acids for each of these proteins. All this code is written by some 25,000 genes. A relatively small number of our genes are permanently turned on and code for our fixed traits, such as skin color, height and other physical attributes. They include a small number of variations that cause so-called single-gene disease. Most genes are inactive and go to work only when called upon, making replacements for worn-out proteins. The resulting proteins perform the functions that express who we are. We need to understand these processes to understand health and illness.

Life is a constant flow of random gene recombinations, experiments so to speak, in an attempt to produce what works the best in the environment. Random errors may occur, thus not every new combination is successful. This means that a gene pool changes slowly over time. Analogous with a computer, a mutant code word can be introduced to replace a less effective one. However, this mechanism does not explain our wide variety of genetic expression.

The Epigenetic Evolution

It turns out that we forgot to look at all the functions of genes. They are subject to a host of regulator genes that read input from the environment and change, not the gene itself, but the genetic messages, depending on the orders they get. This is the power of epigenetics. In addition, they may combine parts from different genes to create patterns to order. These patterns are oftentimes remembered and passed on throughout generations. They explain the infinite nuance and diversity that can arise from our limited number of genes. They can mute an expression, turn on part of a gene or combine snippets. Genes most often work in teams this way. The combined possibilities of this mechanism are practically endless. Diabetes, cardiac disease and most other chronic illnesses have been traced to epigenetics. This tells us that our life is an ongoing reading and incorporation of our environment.

In the end it seems that perhaps both Darwin and Lamarck were a little right for the following reason: Most principles and qualities in nature exhibit dualism, meaning their properties can be taken to extremes in two opposed aspects. Nature tends to avoid extremes, settling into a balance between them. We know this principle from philosophy to physics. Aristotle studied nature and pointed out this balance between the extremes as a harmony that he called "the golden mean." The concepts of "good" and "bad" are not pure in nature. As an often-quoted example, life might be better lived in a balance between excess and deficiency. In philosophy, the idea of the mean might be golden, but it is at work in nature as a mathematical phenomenon called probability distribution.

Events cluster around a central tendency or mean on the so-called bell curve, named for its shape. The probability for a given set of events clusters around the central dome of the curve. Tapering numbers on either side, forming a slope, illustrate the higher and lower probability of the event happening as the curve tapers toward the baseline on either side.

For instance, traits from fear of heights to artistic ability are distributed on this curve.

Nature Is Bell Curved

This infers the idea that randomness is not all that random and can help us better understand the distribution of illness in a population. When epidemiologists and researchers look at human properties in large populations, they find genetic traits such as the propensity toward certain illnesses distributed on the bell curve. We also call it the normal curve because this expresses a normal distribution in a group. Most illness is polygenic, and most of us make up the middle dome of the curve. This represents that most of us can live a healthy life if we take care of ourselves.

As we move toward the tapering edges, we see on the one side increasing propensity toward illness, meaning we have to take good care not to activate gene combinations to make us ill. At the very end of the taper, we find the so-called pure single-gene diseases. The other side tails out in more and more resistant individuals, endowed with an iron health that is literally hard to destroy. The healthy end of the

curve is not salvation. Nor does the illness-prone end represent punishment by the divine hand for sins in a past life. Both are expressions
of nature's variants. A few versions of its designs are unsuccessful.
Luckily, they account for an estimated 5 percent of pathology. The
larger the group, the more accurate the bell curve. Natural selection
acts, not on the individual gene, but on populations. The point is,
this is statistics, not built-in punishment.

We have the knowledge and capacity to skew the curve either
way. We can let natural distribution run its course or skew the curve
to drive genetic activity in our favor or disfavor. With respect to our
health, we have certainly managed to skew it toward illness.

Once we understand genes as servants and tools rather than
masters of our fate, we have to rethink things at a cellular level. If
the wisdom and intelligence to run our lives is not encoded in our
genes and they are merely patterns, then who decides what genes
we use? In other words, who calls upon the genes to make decisions
about health, life and death? Why are so many of us sick that the bell
curve is skewed toward illness? Modern science provides evidence of
behavioral and environmental effects in our health that we have not
yet absorbed.

Meanwhile genetic determinism lives on. We are unable to
rethink the role of genes from causal to consequential, and we don't
think we can change our lives very much. If you have a medical
problem, blame it on your genes. In fact, some of my patients so
adamantly held to their genes as the source of all things ill that they
would take offense at someone trying to take their bad genes from
them! I often hear in conversation, "But you can't escape your genes."
The fallacy is that most of us don't need to escape our genes; we just
need to respect them; some of us a little more than others. Our lack
of understanding of this keeps our entire culture from finding its true
place in the cosmos.

We are not born to be ill.

This is borne out by the new business of human gene analysis,
which at first was thought to be a great tool for finding inherited

health risks. For dearth of such identifiable genes, the study turned to that of ancestry, thereby collecting vast amounts of data. These can be useful in the service of ongoing advanced research on gene fragments.

Quite to the contrary, we have both the genes and the information to maintain good health, yet we are pleading ignorance and waiting for science to come up with the silver bullets to fix us. Medicine tends to avoid looking ahead with "We need more studies." The reality is, we are a long way toward understanding the body in health and illness if we accept the available science.

It has not been all too long since we were thought to consist of blood, bile and phlegm. We have learned anatomy, physiology and biochemistry, allowing us to describe our organ functions and systems. We understand the makeup of our bodies as neatly laid out in cells and molecules at microscopic levels, much like a set of Lego pieces. We have made wonderful progress in high-tech medicine and do amazing lifesaving procedures, including repair of traumatic injury and removal of diseased tissue. Yet there is one problem: these interventions do not reverse disease-producing cellular processes.

Finding the Fountain of Cure

In particular, when it comes to chronic conditions, from which up to some 2/3 of us suffer, we show limited understanding of their origin and meager results in treating them. We offer palliative treatments and flood the body with potions, pills and remedies that mask symptoms. Meanwhile, the processes continue, requiring ever more remedies. While we now understand the connections between our health and many of the more obvious environmental influences such as nutrition and other environmental stresses, this is not where we concentrate our efforts. In fact, in an almost tone-deaf manner we squabble and vilify each other when the discussion turns to the obvious measures we as a society need to take to eradicate these triggers. Instead we continue to put our stock, so to speak, in ever-stronger and better remedies to prop up our failing health. This does prop up stock portfolios while society as a whole struggles with bad health and high insurance costs.

For instance, years ago I took part in a medical delegation to the California legislature to plead the case for stopping the sale of cigarettes to minors. Incredulously, we were told that this particular year was bad for state revenue, and any measures lowering cigarette sales would have to wait!

I am unaware of any medical delegation aiming to stop sugar from being peddled. A few gutsy politicians have tried, but ended up in conflict with industry and without medical backing.

Medicine has built up an enormous system of profit centers around the palliation of symptoms. The management and judgment of the flow of new information is traditionally controlled by monopolies vested in prestige, position and money. Ideas that challenge the status quo may be met with anything from indifference to hostility and even persecution, as this is an easy way to protect hegemony and control against "heretics and crackpots." It also absolves the power structure from open-minded consideration and scientific scrutiny of new ideas.

This has led to costly delays of much groundbreaking advancements because these are often counterintuitive and hidden from our view and immediate understanding.

Furthermore, by its very nature of unmeasurables, medicine is not considered a hard-core science, but rather, as so poetically expressed in medical training, "an art and a science." Its history is one of empirical observations often tinted by fads, philosophy, personal bias, prejudice and commercialism. We have been prescribed anything from blood-letting to mercury with no understanding of their deleterious effects. We are now being lulled into thinking that new interventions will "heal" us. This has led to an erosion of trust in orthodox medicine as seen by the mushrooming of alternative healing. Unfortunately, not even this type of medicine quite fathoms how we need to adopt the understanding of biological systems implied by the last hundred years of scientific discovery. This understanding is key to the global concept of human health. Once we shift our view here, we can begin to set up a different paradigm.

The Blind Leading the Blind?

In an almost delusional manner, there is an industry of ambitious initiatives to look through the microscope for the fountain of wellness, that is, efforts to "stamp out" or "end all illness" through million-dollar study projects. We insist on spending billions in laboratories looking at cells while we are missing the point. We are looking for high-tech miracles to bend nature while we fail to understand that we function at its pleasure as an integral part of the universe. Only understanding this will truly give us choices. We can consciously choose to be well or sick. This book looks at the forces that make it so.

As these connections continue to elude us, what makes us ill is stumbling in front of us while we stare down our ailing bodies. We will come up long on money and, sadly, short on results.

So here we are, the surviving fittest, sitting on top of the globe in all our glory, living out our outdated phantasy. Meanwhile, science tells us that we are part of a universal flow of energy clinging on to a brittle, tenuous surface of a planet that is racing through space at one thousand miles per hour. We are totally at its mercy because we are interdependent. Our very survival is a function of this relationship. We are cosmic in nature, and the planet is our source and mirror. It gives us back what we ask for. The universe is the ultimate model of a holistic system.

Right here let us pause a minute to gather our thoughts around the word "holistic." It has become so overused that it is worth rethinking its true meaning: it implies a whole entity made up of multiple integrated components that derive their significance from being part of the whole.

We can make our journey here as good or as bad as we wish by how well we understand this. If you now are totally mystified and confused, thinking this is a lesson in philosophy, let us start by stepwise developing our cosmic model from the individual cell.

The Incredible Cell

The smallest independent unit of life is the single cell. We forget it, but this is the cell from whence we came. Ours is called eukaryotic because it has a kernel or nucleus that houses our genes. It also contains the vestiges of all our vital organs in little enclosures called organelles (little organs). Their very names are our clues that they can perform all the functions of the body. The single cell can live independently and reacts appropriately to its surroundings. It reads the environment, moves to seek nurturing while recognizing old and new threats, seeking to avoid them while defending itself if need be. In short, the single cell shows awareness of its environment and solves problems; all measures of intelligence. All without a separate brain.

Evolutionarily, the cell discovered that there is strength in numbers and started banding together with others; not a bad idea. A slime mold is just that to us. It has no brain, but below our radar it creates a home and lives a purposeful life. It negotiates mazes, choses a balanced diet; in fact, it shows altruistic behavior in times of food shortage. We could now proceed by adding morphology, and the slug appeared. Next came the realization that if some cells took over one function, this would strengthen the whole and free up others to specialize in something else, and we started developing limbs and other organs to improve our efficiency.

Too bad we are too advanced to see this. From using the skin as our sensory organ, we developed specialized cells such as eyes and ears and pipelines of conduction for the signals we picked up, known as nerves, leading to the brain.

The sum of this development is, of course, the human body, some seventy trillion cells messaging to the brain, which interprets, processes and responds. The perfect organization of all components, all valuable and useful, makes us the most sophisticated and complex of all beings on this planet. We could not function optimally without the cooperation of all those integral parts because the system is holistic. We are all better off when everyone has a place and mission. It seems that we would honor ourselves by taking our cues from this amazing design. Not understanding this lesson keeps us out of the universal loop. In fact, so much so that we are losing links of our holistic chain by the day.

We are Physical Beings

Our cells are made of organic materials, mostly a collection of proteins surrounded by a membrane made of fat and cholesterol. The bulk of our working cells consists of hundreds of thousands of proteins that make up our structure and function. The nucleus contains our genetic information or genome. The cell proteins have been called the bearers of life because they bring instructions to the genes to form building blocks and elements that code for our lives. They include hundreds of thousands of specialized proteins working in relay as messengers, effectors, binding agents, enzymes, hormones and catalysts in constant communication with each other and the outside. In short, they are the network of pathways for most body processes. We think of this as a Newtonian or mechanical engine working in linear order, explained by molecular structures and chemical energy transfers. However, this idea falls short, and things get complicated fast.

We are Electrical Beings

First off, what drives these processes? We need a reliable fuel source. The food we eat has thermal or heat energy measured in calories, but we cannot sprinkle food on a muscle to make it move. This immediately reminds us that the body's energy production is a lengthy and involved process.

Energy Metabolism

Food stuffs are heat energy or calories transformed into chemical power by a reaction called the Krebs cycle, followed by the so-called respiratory cycle. To enter this transformation, all foodstuffs must be sugar or sugar-like molecules, here called sugars for short. It turns sugar into chemical energy molecules known as ATP or adenosine triphosphate.

Here is where it gets interesting: The energy of ATP is used to separate positively and negatively charged ions such as sodium, chloride, potassium and hydrogen ions called electrolytes across the cell wall to create a charge or voltage.

If this is beginning to sound like your car battery, you are right. We are battery driven, and the power source is sugar. This voltage potential is fundamental to our cell functioning, and sensitive to changes in the environment

The strength of this voltage depends partly on our electrolyte and acid-base balance. Our cells hold their charge and function best in a weakly alkaline environment and at a certain balance among electrolytes. Any shift toward acidity or electrolyte imbalance will lower the voltage across the cell wall, predisposing us to illness. In fact, if we lost our charge we would die.

The processing from food to life-sustaining electricity is our energy metabolism. The biochemistry and physics involved here can be described and measured. Don't laugh; science is actually looking at ways to use our electrical power to run small gadgets.

The cells go through this entire process just to produce the electric energy to run our life. But how does electricity become action? This is done by a different, even more complex signaling system that directs our behavior.

To understand it, we must enter the realm of electromagnetics, even brush up against quantum physics.

We can simplify by dividing it into steps.

Proteome Power

The cell proteins are arranged in a web, almost like a tangled ball of yarn, called the proteome. This maze of pathways is activated by the messages or signals that direct biological behavior.

The proteome pathways are unpredictable and unmeasurable in physical terms. A does not simply lead to B. It can lead to B, D, C, X, Z, to all, to some, or travel in reverse. They can switch the message on or off, intertwine or integrate, amplify or diminish it, reroute or block it. In addition, the networks are redundant and can be used for different messages.

We can now appreciate that interpreting human physiology in light of classical physics is one of our fallacies, because, as we shall see, such a linear system would fail to explain the behavior of the message as well as the result.

We are at the doorstep of quantum theory. Fear not, all we need to understand for our purposes is the very basics of its role in energy flow. We have not yet internalized this fundamental concept and its consequences.

Signal Transduction

Picture each cell membrane totally covered by antennae. They are called receptors, and their job is in the name. They detect and pick up signals or messages from the environment. The signals latch on to a designated receptor and depolarize the cell membrane, releasing its energy. It is used to start the cellular process of transforming any signal into electrical impulses that travel through the maze of the proteome pathways that we just described. Here we meet another amazing function of proteins: in the moist cell environment they exist as charged particles that are excellent electrical conductors. The process is called transduction, referring to the amazing change taking place, and the pathways are aptly called "transduction pathways." Based on their nature and mission, the signals are led through the pathways and enter the nucleus where they find their target genes or trigger for their designated forms of biological work. The signals can come as one, in layers or in multiples.

The process is called an electro-conformational change. It is a multi-energy conversion process because the original signal can be any from a sound to a hormone. The interaction of the signal with the cell may cause changes anywhere throughout the system. However, the messages are nuanced as our behavior, and here is how that comes about:

We are Electronic Beings

If we give our electricity a language to work with, we can create very complicated actions. We can do this because the proteome actually functions as a transistor, funneling the signals through a selective electronic circuitry.

If you work with computers, you might recognize the principle here.

The input comes from the outside. The signal being transmitted is information that becomes integrated in the form of electrical charges. In the tech world, this might be called the signal-transduction pathways in informational technology.

Paraphrasing a quote ascribed to Intel: "Signals converge, integrate and become electrical energy somewhere along this network. Signal transduction circuits in biological systems have molecular on/off switches that, like those in a computer chip, thus transmit information when on."

The cell receptor is the keyboard, the signal transduction happens in the transducer, and our central processing unit is the cell. Body cells are capable of processing information about everyday autonomous functioning, but the more complicated processing work goes through the ultimate processor—the brain. When the signal reaches its target, the final readout is the biological work intended by the original signal and executed accordingly by the body. The cell is our personal computer!

It is key and this cannot be overstated: we program our body from the outside on an ongoing basis with information we take down from the environment. We function on information. The programming depends on what signals or first messengers we choose.

We Are Electromagnetic Beings

All of our cells produce electricity, but the cells of our muscles, nervous and endocrine system all operate at the higher voltages, meaning they produce stronger currents. Currents radiate energy waves called electromagnetic fields. These are fields of information that affect cellular function and maintain our health. They can be measured as, for instance, electrocardiograms and electroencephalograms. Perturbances of the normal field may lead to weakening of the body.

We explained earlier that increasing acidity lowers the voltage across the cell membrane and thus weakens the current and electromagnetic field. Changes in ions and acidity will change the current, thus the electromagnetic field and the message. These findings might be more than coincidence, since a basic feature of chronic illness is increased acidity.

To get the full picture of our "animal magnetism"—by the way, that is no joke—we now need to move our discussion to the atomic or quantum level. First to the atomic nucleus. It is made up of moving particles that move or spin. We are all in constant motion, spontaneously creating waves of energy in the form of local magnetic fields so weak they are barely registrable. Every organ has its own nuclear spin frequency. This spin energy can be augmented or diminished by outside energy, creating either resonance or dissonance and determining the energy balance of the system. We use the energy of magnetic resonance (MRI) for obtaining diagnostic imagery of the body.

We Light Up the Room

In addition, we emit other energies, including light, spontaneously. Well, not normal light, but an ultra-weak light energy called biophotons that are measured in units of quanta. They vibrate to resonate at certain frequencies with cells and organisms. This corresponds to certain functions involved with the regulation of energy and information transfer in the body. Biophotons are shown to increase during stress. Their optimal functioning is essential to health.

Like their stronger counterparts that we just mentioned, the waves communicate with other fields, matter and energies and have been shown to impact our entire life cycle including growth and development by carrying information between tissues, organs and the outside world. In particular, they are important influences on the immune system. Consequently, if perturbed, they are most effective in disrupting our health. Our complex biological behavior is attached to the health of our energy fields.

We Are Quantum Beings

Atoms are too small to observe with the naked eye or the microscope, too elusive to measure with sticks and tapes, and the fundamental concept is that at this level, matter and wave are interchangeable forms of energy.

We are now in quantum territory, and the full weight, so to speak, of this idea comes with the electrons. They are weightless and move so fast that they appear as clouds. Quantum theory defines them as waves, but also as particles; well, not even particles, but by probability of where they can be found. Describing them must be done, not by location, but by mathematics. Furthermore, quantum tells us that our experience of things is uncertain and depends on how we observe them. All this cannot be explained by classical physics, and introduces quantum uncertainty. This is more than theory, as we saw in the principle of the proteome. Weird isn't it?

The final weird idea we must touch on is the entanglement of energies. Energies can read and change each other over distance. Our ability to connect this way has been called quantum spookiness.

Minding Our Ps and Qs: The Proteome Is a Quantum Concept

Let us look again at the path of the traveling signal. Remember, the proteome can effect the transduction of matter to energy and energy to matter. The pathways are unpredictable, making the outcome uncertain.

This has consequences: when we present any unknown form of energy to our body, the outcome is not linear but uncertain. It could offer surprises, and it does, as we will see later.

Another one bites the dust: We have held to the idea that quantum phenomena are only theoretical ideas at subatomic level. What we have just said is that quantum mechanics are alive and well at the level of our body molecules right under our noses so to speak, working hand in hand with our known molecular forces. And the result is the seamless functioning that is us. We are indeed quantum beings.

The Human Energy Field

Here is the point of all this:

Adding up the forces we have discussed, we now have a network of particle-waves that affect the state of the body and the mind through electrical and quantum energies that meld together. When all parts of the system vibrate to create an integrated wave, they produce a unique or signature energy of the individual. This is called biomagnetism, collectively constituting the human energy field. Healthy cells show strong energy fields, which again promote a healthy body. Perturbances to any part of the field may lead to dysfunction or illness.

You might recall from high-school physics that waves of the same wavelength amplify each other. Positive amplifies the wave and negative; you get the picture. We assign value to energy commensurate with its effects on our health. We call this energy template perception.

By definition, if we find a stimulus to be positive, it resonates with our positive energy and reinforces our well-being. Conversely, an injury will induce an injury current, and the field will change accordingly.

Our signature energy field defines us, including our homeostasis or usual state of the body, and any perturbance to the body may derange the field.

Long-standing stress, age and disease may weaken the field and be dangerous to our health. Energy fields can influence the function of our immune cells, affecting our ability to fight disease.

This is not just a theoretical concept. Above we mentioned negative energy in the form of fear. Mental energy at stress levels alerts the nervous system to start stress hormone production, the first step in alerting the immune system. If it goes on, we may see heart attacks, ulcers and other "stress-diseases." We call these psychosomatic diseases without really thinking of what goes into them. They are created by ambient negative energy. Careful what you wish for and who you commune with!

We use the term injury current in the service of medicine. We can, in fact, measure the electromagnetic fields at the site of bony injuries. The field force we register is called an injury current. Likewise, we use what we call healing current to treat them. We see the normalization of the field as the bone heals. It is of note that not all manner of injury is thought to respond. Electromagnetic waves are used in the treatment of some forms of mental illness, though more gently and wisely than the old high energy electroshock method, which was injurious rather than healing. Learning to understand energy can give us advantages where we need them.

Magnetic fields have no borders and are not limited to specific areas. All electrically charged elements in the universe similarly produce electromagnetic fields of information, and interact with our biofield. We are part of this larger energy flow.

Melding together, the sum of these energies becomes the cosmic flow of energy that connects us with each other and weaves us into the flow of the universe, reflecting our health and the overall health of the universe.

We spend our lives reading and emitting incoming electromagnetic waves, adding our waves to the conversation. This is the reception and broadcast of our universe and the ultimate expression of our holistic nature. The entire body is, in effect, a biological and an electronic engine integrated in the cosmic flow of energy. We are conversant with e-mail, e-bikes, e-commerce and the like. Well, we are e-people and we are on the internet!

A couple of simple examples: Have you ever been in a room with persons and felt their aura before you ever saw their face or talked to them, or walked into an apparently empty house and known someone was there? You were reading energy fields.

Everything Is Energy, or Energy Is Everything

Since all of us are part of the energy flow, energies of the same character and wave lengths would reinforce each other. We call it resonance. Our health depends on the part of the flow to which we are exposed. Furthermore, our choices will have an impact throughout the system.

We become "one with" what we connect with. We may say that our health and that of the universe are the continuous integration of this energy, the essence of holism. This is a good time to repeat the definition of holism: the comprehension of all parts of a system interconnected into an indivisible whole.

Oops, whatever happened to Newton's physical reality? Is everything simply what we can see and touch? And what has magnetism to do with my cells? And my life?

As you can see, a lot. Biological systems are quantum systems in perpetual flux between matter and wave. This equilibrium keeps changing with how we interact with the universe. The incoming signals are the information that change the energy field. The closer we keep the exchange to our signature biofield, the healthier we are.

We are constantly bombarded by possibilities from which we chose. Once we bring things into consciousness they may collapse into particles and enter the physical world. While this might seem a little like explaining the biblical transformation of water to wine, we can comprehend holism, which in reality is a quantum concept.

Quantum theory is difficult to apprehend, and it has stayed more or less in the scientific shadows. The most common popular interpretation is expressed in self-help books referring to this universal energy as "vibes" and asserting that pressing your nose up against the shop window and wishing—that is, using instant "creating your new reality"—the pearls on display can be yours! The missing piece here is that the observer-created reality is a mathematical feature of the quantum world. It is not a linear relation between cause and effect in the specific case; rather, it is the expression of intent or shifting focus to open up new pathways or probabilities that might lead to the desired result.

This level of understanding came to us during the first part of the last century. Some one hundred years ago, a cadre of bright young physicists took the next leap to bring us into the world of electromagnetism, leading to modern physics and quantum theory, changing our understanding of our world.

This science of uncertainty might come as overwhelming news to you, but don't feel alone. A certain fellow named Albert Einstein, while helping to create it, objected to the loss of determinism implied in quantum theory. If matter is a wave and vice versa, and if their nature is a question of how we perceive them, then the management has been taken out of the divine hand. Determinism is gone and nothing is certain. If you find this disconcerting, so did he. However, no new theories have replaced this view.

Biology—Molecular or Quantum?

We now have alternate ways to describe living systems. The physical organism can be seen as molecules, and organs that can be measured and counted. Its functioning is explained by anatomy and chemical reactions. When a system is seen on this scale, we see it as classic. Our health is assessed by physical exams and tests.

On the other hand, our physical bodies meld with, in fact, can be described as energy fields exchanging information to create and maintain health. We exist in both dimensions and are subject to the laws of both. We can simply think of it as holistic biology.

Modern physicists and other scientists who have long felt that human energy fields are fundamental to health have been ignored, if not ridiculed. It is a pleasure to announce that mavericks like Drs. Makela, Liboff, and others were vindicated with a 2008 article in *Science Daily*, reporting that "magnetism has been used to trigger cellular reactions normally induced by drugs or hormones."

This stunning piece of scientific progress went largely under the radar.

The ideas here rely heavily on modern physics, and seem lofty and remote to medicine, firmly rooted in its familiar physical language. They could also potentially cause conflict of interest with the drug industry, which guards its territory assiduously.

While no one has yet arrived at a unifying theory between the linear physics of large-scale objects and quantum physics, the body shows no conflict integrating the two dimensions. If we took our cues from the body we might come up with an integrated view of our health where molecules and energy fields cooperate.

The real issue may be our lack of understanding of the origins of illness. If we miss looking through the quantum lens, we are left in the Newtonian world, leaving us outside the universal flow of energy. Ignoring the integrated nature of our cellular processes we miss the results.

Meanwhile, medicine wonders about the next "quantum leap." Quantum indeed.

Why have we gone through this lengthy journey of explaining the functioning of our cells? Because, as you can see, the dimension of energy in health and medicine is no longer a far-flung philosophical idea. Science can account for the phenomena at work, even integrate them. Many people look to understand these connections, and the information should be available to us all. This field is obviously in its infant stages, and there is a lot of work to be done to determine its role and utility.

If you believe in the role of energy in disease and healing, you might have encountered some skepticism. Science has spoken: You were right all along.

The Cell Should Keep Us Safe

Sadly, medical doctrine operates in the world of the mechanical cell and the linear process. This view implies that we might have reached the end of development of medicine because there is little reason to think cells can learn to integrate and problem-solve.

The whole point of this chapter has been to bear witness to what science already has told us: the cell reasons. Dumb? I respectfully refer to the plethora of research we have drawn on already.

The next dead-end argument by medicine is that if cells were intelligent, we could teach them how to repair themselves in case of injury. Since we cannot, they must be dumb? But cells replace their old worn-out parts constantly. Hello? For the most part, cells are not in need of replacement parts; they are poisoned by negative energies.

Speaking of replacement parts, we are unwilling to accept that we exist here a limited time in this form, then we join the eternal universal energy flow in a different one. We want to take ourselves out of this cosmic cycle, oh, and redesign our species to be the one that lives forever with lab-grown or harvested parts. Hello?

Our idea of progress seems to aim at teaching our cells to rejuvenate us and to right all our wrongs.

This way we might live forever without taking care of ourselves while ordering our cells to fix it. It would then follow, for instance, that cigarette-smoking would not be harmful to the "trained" cell. Reckless living is a curious definition of intelligence. We refuse to give the cell what it needs to be healthy, and therefore it is dumb? It is almost an embarrassment of riches to ask who is dumb here. Can we abdicate responsibility for ourselves, or does our understanding and behavior need to be part of the solution?

We are also putting our faith in gene therapy. The problem is that since so many proclivities towards illnesses are polygenetic (determined by many genes), we might have to redesign our entire genome, literally rein-vent ourselves, to avoid them.

These stumbling blocks have us thinking we have reached "the end of the development of medicine." Worse yet, it has us failing to think we can realign ourselves with the forces that shape us. We might do well to rethink these ideas.

The Intelligent Cell

If you have learned anything so far, it should be awe of the genius of our population of seventy trillion cells. Inundated with the constant cosmic bombardment of ideas, it came up with us. Not to mention being hard at work 24-7 making highly complex decisions to manage, protect and defend us. We are reluctant to give up our humancentric ideas of other life-forms being dumb and brainless.

In reality we are the dumb and brainless who don't understand the language, customs and home of whales, ravens, frogs, or amoebae. Much as we think we have a monopoly on "civilization," we don't understand them because we only see the world from our perspective. Speaking of civilization, ours has shown itself brutal beyond anything seen in the animal world. Our failure to understand our connectedness is destroying their home, and in the end, our own.

Living cells function on what is taken down from the universe and presented to them. Every one of our intelligent, hardworking cells is waiting for the next thing coming at them. What am I going to be exposed to? Inhaling smoke? A pound of candy? Will I be allowed to thrive or made to fight? We are big boys and girls. Our health decisions are not made by the cells; they are made by how we choose to treat them. Let that sink in.

What Starts this Process?

By now you have a whole new understanding how we align with the universe, and we saved the best for last: what kind of signals initiate the path of the signal-transduction pathway of informational metabolism?

First, let us look a little closer at the receptor cells that make up the keyboard. Recall that the body is a sponge of antennae that pick up the faintest signal from the environment. They enter through skin, mucus membranes, every orifice in the body and, above all, through the sensory organs to the brain.

The receptors or antennae perceive and interpret these signals from sound, touch, vision, toxins, smell, hearing, love, danger, stress and trauma in the context of culture and emotions. They all find their designated receptor that helps them enter the pathway.

Key here is that any form of energy, be it wave or matter, good or bad, that makes contact with any receptor on any of our cells is a signal or first messenger, is funneled into the cell. There it engages the proteins and genes related to its ultimate biological expression or function. It may be fine-tuned by hormones, enzymes or other modifiers. The cells also use internal signals to communicate with each other.

At the end these messages, for good or for bad, change the cell and write the script of our lives at that moment.

Our Choices Shape Us

We, the die-hard exceptionalists, are becoming more and more isolated from each other and from nature. We miss the order and expression of purpose that occurs at every level in nature and in organisms with or without a brain. We are suffering from a disconnect that we don't quite understand. It now is being recognized as lack of exposure to others and to nature.

Even trees and rocks take down the information to communicate internally and with their neighbors in this actualization of possibilities. It becomes a shared observation. The participants agree on the meaning of this information and create a community.

We are in This Together

As we maneuver through this world of endless possibilities, we must become holistic thinkers because no person or action is separated from the whole. The ultimate consequence of a choice will eventually come back to visit us, other parts of our universe or those who follow us. The more we understand the consequence of our choices, the wiser they will be. With our limited perspective we might not see it, but it is implied. This might also give us pause to look at what we have created so far. Our health can be seen as a metaphor for it. It also determines the quality of our lives.

Once we understand this connectedness, we begin to take down positive energy such as empathy and harmony with our co-travelers and the planet. We are in this together. Spiritual and healing observances are those that reinforce our holistic nature and our connectedness. We become quantum thinkers. Our fate is not predetermined.

Neither is our health. We create and shape both with what parts of this we call into the pathway.

By taking care of the whole we are indeed the creators of our own destiny.

Many of our forebears intuitively sensed it. They understood that consciousness is not necessarily attached to brains or thoughts. They perceived a cosmic flow where everything in nature has intent and purpose in the larger scheme of things. Leonardo da Vinci noted to the point that "everything is connected in a great system in perpetual movement." Much to our peril we call this recognition of the cosmic energy flow "primitive," "new wave," or worse. We are missing the larger connectedness. Understanding our true nature confers power, but also responsibility for the welfare of the whole.

Redefining Health

The World Health Organization states that good health is not merely the absence of illness, but the state of complete physical, mental and social well-being. While this describes the perfect state of affairs, it does not give us any clues as to what goes into this state or how to maintain it.

All our life-giving processes are signals from the universe, without which we would not exist. We have just redefined our health to include the carefully coded information of the entire environment that informs our lives. The constant stream of information we take down from the universe into our cells creates the energy state that is our life and health.

We can say so without reservation, because without this activity, our lives could not happen.

We cannot tune in to these basic principles, neither can we find answers as long as we respond to this information by shooting the messengers.

We will spend this book elucidating how matter and energy affects the balance of our own, well, matter or energy!

So let us look at our incredible body that takes us through this journey, whether we accept it or not.

CHAPTER 2
How the Body Works

We Are Wired for Efficiency

While this is an enormous topic, we will concentrate on the most important organ systems that pertain to our discussion.

We are the perfect network of organs wired for efficiency of communication linked by a major conduit called the endocrine system. It directs biology by producing a plethora of messenger molecules that intertwine with physical and electrical conduction systems, the most prominent being the circulatory and the nervous system. Together they are important long-distance carriers of nutrients and information throughout the body and beyond.

The Endocrine System

This system includes nerve cells and glands that produce hormones. These are small molecules produced and distributed throughout the brain and body that interchange with a cadre of other messengers, tissues and organs to direct our physical as well as psychological and emotional states. Expressed differently, the system includes electrically powered cells influenced by the environment to produce particles that influence our energy state. It literally negotiates changes of our thoughts and mood by changing the flux of energy between matter and wave.

The Cardiovascular System

Fueled by electricity, the heart functions as the perpetual central pump, working off a charge called a rolling electric potential. We can only live for a few minutes without the action of this pump because it is responsible for our oxygen supply.

The consequence of interruption in electric signaling may be grave. The heart starts skipping beats. It needs to be efficient and responsive, delivering blood to the body in proportions to changing needs through tubing we call vessels. How much our heart needs to work and the regulation of flow in the vessels are very tightly regulated by the diverse agents mentioned above: nerves, hormones, neurotransmitters and other chemicals. If we look closer at these regulators, they mostly find their origin in the environment. Our production of hormones, such as adrenalin and cortisone, fluctuate in response to our surroundings, even time of day or available light.

The Nervous System

The nervous system is a tangle of tubing of sensory cells throughout all corners of the body carrying complex information quickly and efficiently. They connect organs of specialized receptor tissue called our senses and the brain. Equipped with acute sensory capacity for the specific stimuli, they are expert at translating energy fast, sometimes instantly. They transact some of our most critical and complex interactions with our environment such as smell, sound, sight, touch and taste.

Signals are sent to the brain, which makes the complex decisions of what to do with incoming information. As with other signals, these systems work on tightly controlled electronic principles to fine-tune the message. The body signals the brain what is going on, and the brain integrates and responds. We depend on this highway of information to function normally.

The Brain

It only makes sense that our enormous community of cells needs a central government. The brain is the CEO, so to speak. This world of some seventy trillion intelligent working individuals is a network of highways carrying information to and from the outside of the body. It does so by using some one hundred billion electrical cells, called neurons, bound in infinitely complicated circuits and pathways that change their connectivity, adding or deleting as we go. We can easily measure and record the brain's electrical signals, as we can those of the heart.

The Secret of Brainpower?

The brain is the central station that collects information from every part of the body and the environment. We are barraged with a flurry of input from everywhere all the time. Luckily, we have a filtering mechanism capable of straining out much of this chaos while retaining what we deem valuable.

The brain is expert at creative thinking and uniquely equipped to override the body cells if need be. We are masters of pattern recognition, learning languages and ideas by recognizing patterns of sound, images and pressure. We memorize by using specialized areas for storing and retrieving incoming images and ideas, comparing new ones with the ones stored in memory.

This pattern-processing gives us the ability to expand on our cognitive framework or reference frame. We transfer and integrate the result of known or perceived patterns to new ones, reworking them into new ideas to upgrade our software, so to speak.

Our mind can apprehend abstractions from the world of infinite possibilities, enabling us to plan, design and implement objects in the actual world. This process is fathomable through the writings by mathematical philosophers such as Whitehead, postulating a realm of possibilities called the metaphysical world. We apprehend and manifest these through our awareness or consciousness.

Like other signals, thoughts are influenced by hormones and signal modulators, many of which are unique to the brain. Nerve cells release transmitter substances that influenc the electric conduction, thus the final shape and character of the signals.

The combination of a large cerebrum, signal modulators and electric energy makes the brain the supercomputer, able to transform signals into complex responses such as our ability for abstraction and creativity.

To appreciate the complexity involved here, we might compare thinking to processing in the binary electronic system of a computer trying to signal a mood. It would take a lot of 1s and 0s! The complicated processing done by the brain is energy-consuming. With some 2 percent of our body weight it accounts for some 20 percent of our energy use.

The Brain Is Linked In

We can easily see that the brain is not the isolated boss in the corner office. It is linked in by its energy called the mind. Modern mathematics point out that it can be defined as an open non-linear integrational system regulating the flow of information among us, meaning that it reaches out of its own space and can cascade or amplify its effects into the environment. Its open nonlinear quality points us to the holistic laws of biological systems.

The mind is a relational process, receiving and returning to its environment; that is, by definition integrating us into the holistic energy flow of the universe. Framed by our ideals and aspirations, our thoughts represent our spiritual values. The regulation of our mind, the collective behavior of cellular systems, can only be understood in terms of its holistic or quantum nature.

The Second Brain.

Before continuing, we must mention a surprise connection. We have another "brain" though an unlikely one: the gut. Our intestine contains trillions of microbes that we call the microbiota. It is closely linked to the brain by a multitude of nerve cells lining its walls. It also contains half of our immune cells. This makes sense since this is the place where an infinite variety of substances enters the body and need to be scrutinized as they enter.

Surprisingly, it also produces many of the neurochemicals found in the brain. This links the brain to the gut in what is called the gut-brain axis, with information flowing in both directions.

The axis is again intimately linked to the immune system in the gut wall. Information flows between the brain and the immune system in a three-way linkage through this intestinal integration.

This stabilizing complex run by microbes could indeed be called the second brain.

A healthy gut flora is key in helping digestion, keeping bad microbes in check and protecting against illness.

While it does not directly help us in learning math, it produces a number of hormones that decrease stress, influence our mood, notably the brain hormone serotonin, and act as an integrating hub for somatic and mental functioning, even facilitating higher functions, such as learning and memory. Keeping our gut flora healthy is vital to the entire body and our immune defenses. It underscores the idea of health as an integrated process. These relatively recently discovered connections are the subject of intense research with respect to disease processes.

Our Formidable Homeland Defense: The Immune System

Now that we have a sense of the flow of information throughout the body, it is time to look at our homeland security.

The body is protected by a formidable defense system. It needs to work on the macro as well as the micro level and be prepared to tackle any challenger at any time. It consists of several multilayered integrated mechanisms collectively known as the immune system. You probably think of this as producing antibodies in response to an illness, but that does not quite cover its scope of action. You can see that producing antibodies would not save us from the jaws of a hungry lion. For large external threats, we need to use quick thinking and muscle to outrun our attacker. As we will see, we have just such a mechanism at our disposal. Whatever the trigger, the immune system has a limited repertoire of responses. In fact, it has one common response that shows a number of variations on a theme: inflammation.

The Fight-or-Flight Reflex

In the 1920s, Dr. Walter Cannon described the trigger of the fight-or-flight response as stress. Revived as a concept in the 1970s by Dr. Hans Seyle, stress has come to mean any psychological or biological challenge to the body's immune system. The National Institute of Mental Health has their version: "the brain's response to any demand."

While we emphasize that mild stress can be motivating, perceived attacks from the environment elicit an instant response mechanism that allows for a quick getaway. We call this the fight-or-flight system. It is a reflex response to fear. On an instant's notice, part of our nervous system starts producing a surge of the stress-hormone adrenalin to shift our metabolism away from daily duties such as digestion. This shunts available calories to the brain and the muscles to make a speedy retreat. We raise our heart rate, increase our breathing and start releasing sugar into the bloodstream to fuel our effort.

In the case of a smaller threat, adrenalin simply puts the rest of the immune system on alert. If the stress continues, a second stress hormone, cortisol, steps in for the long haul. It works by funneling resources into the fight. In the case of sustained stress, cortisol starts funneling resources to the immune system. It breaks down muscle protein and converts it to sugar, promotes muscle and bone loss and raises blood sugar while depositing unused calories as fat around the body, leading to atrophy of limbs and central weight gain. This constant alert actually may exhaust the immune system. These are reasons why prolonged stress is not good for us.

Inflammation

Classic inflammation is a standard response first described around the first century BC and is still true: redness, pain, swelling, fever and decreased function, depending on the severity of stress. It is the body's response to severe or sustained threats, whether they be high-energy wave or matter-related, and it unfolds in layers.

The purpose of this reaction is to drive out the negative energy, whatever its nature, and restore order. This underscores the importance of understanding our discussion of our lives as a flow of different forms of energy. We now have a new definition of good health: the absence of negative energy to avoid triggering inflammation.

Not all inflammation comes with a fanfare. In fact, most of it is stealth, low-grade stressors that insinuate themselves onto—not to say into—our bodies, oftentimes without us recognizing them as stressors. The chronic response is correspondingly low grade. It might be invisible to the eye, but we might register an elevated blood sugar, blood pressure, a wheezing or an indigestion. Our immune system is now working in low gear. There is a certain steal going on from the body to boost the immune system, and we are not at our best.

We Cannot Be in Two Places at One Time

All told, the immune system is comprised of the part of the nervous system as well as cells found all over our body including in our bone marrow, spleen, lymph nodes, tonsils and gut.

When there are no threats, we are in positive energy and the immune system is inactive. Our focus can go toward building ourselves up. We call that anabolic or *thrive* phase. Conversely, a threat will put the body in negative or *defense* mode. We really cannot multitask, and so it is in either mode at the expense of its other systems and organs, which quickly redirect their resources accordingly. Just think of how you feel if you have a simple cold. Energy starts flowing into healing, and we feel tired. If the attacker persists, the inflammatory process may go on permanently at a stalemate. This may mean an ongoing repair process, causing a high turnover of cells.

These two phases are coordinated by a cadre of hormone-like substances that act much like an on-off switch on the immune system, directing resources to where they are needed. In the long run it may stunt growth, even kill us. Any negative energy can trigger the immune system and may lead to physical or mental illness.

Stressors Come in All Grades

We can divide stressors into infectious and non-infectious ones. The non-infectious ones are non-live irritants and toxins in the environment. They could be edibles, breathables, thoughts (yes, you read it right) or overuse of muscles. They represent low grade exposure to things we don't tolerate and will cause us ill effects in the long run. They may fester in silence for years before they cause us real problems.

Responses Come in Layers

Faced with a subacute irritant, our innate immune system is called upon to deal with it. The basic mechanism starts at the lowest step and adjusts upward in layers of response as an illness unfolds.

Layer

A message goes to the nervous system to start producing adrenalin. If the threat is large and fast, the muscle is recruited. If the intruder gets under the skin, adrenalin switches on the genes to produce inflammatory cells and toxins that circulate in the blood to locate and kill the bum. This is known as the innate immune system. It activates a series of cells throughout the body and particularly around openings to the environment such as the lungs and the gastrointestinal tract, where intruders are likely to attack. They are literally detectives and customs inspectors all at once. All visitors are scrutinized.

Remember that the gut is our largest customs station because about half of our immune cells are stationed along the gastric tract, eyeing the endless stream of old and new incoming substances. The good guys get a pass, but the moment a suspicious agent enters the body, it is reported to the immune system, which starts mobilizing a collection of large ferocious cells called macrophages or killer cells (meaning they are large and eat anything!) and other cells whose mission is self-explanatory. For good measure, they also spew out a variety of immune modifiers and toxins. Many body cells can be recruited and can transform into macrophage-like cells to join the fight. If this is not enough, the immune system has plenty of resources to draw from.

- upon Layer

The cell walls in the affected area activate the so-called eicosanoid system that influences inflammation by releasing substances called omega-3 and omega-6. These are fatty acids with unusual properties. Omega-3 is anti-inflammatory; in fact, it gives a boost to wellness in the normal cell while the second type, omega-6, competes with omega-3 for the cell receptor and displaces it. From there it can release more inflammatory agents. A healthy body depends on a good ratio of omega-3 to 6. We cannot synthesize either, thus we depend on nutrition to keep a healthy balance. Omega-6 is abundant while omega-3 is less available.

- upon Layer

We are now aware of a substance of ancient origin found in most body cells all through the phylogenetic tree called ubiquitin. It is our earliest known defense system found even in single cell organisms and still very much with us. It runs another system of starting and stopping inflammation, including the so-called ubiquitin proteasome pathway that cleans up the inflammatory protein debris left on the battlefield of inflammatory reactions as they resolve. This system is activated in inflammation of any cause.

- upon Layer

At this point we need to make the acquaintance of a special set of immune receptors called human leucocyte antigens, or HLA receptors. These are specialized protein receptors that recognize our cells as "ours." Without these receptors, the immune system would not know the difference between your tissue and mine; we could literally be anyone.

While they were first discovered in high numbers in the immune system, they are present on most of our cells. They scrutinize all substances reaching our tissues. This way, if a cell or protein displaying non-self HLA receptors shows up, cells located almost anywhere in the body can easily sound the alarm and turn into fighters anytime, and the newcomer is resoundingly attacked. This is one of the problems of human organ transplantation. In that scenario, we call the protection of self a transplant rejection.

The real lesson here is consistent with what we have learned so far: the information to make us unique is not in our cells; it is in the receptors. And remember, the receptors by themselves do nothing until they receive and transmit information from the outside into the cell. An outside substance has to show up for the HLA receptor to show its magic and recognize our uniqueness. This drives home a major point: our unique "self" comes from the outside world.

- upon Layer

Thus far we have looked at our innate defense mechanisms against non-live intruders.

Live pathogens like bacteria, viruses and other invaders may take up residence in our cells and use them as incubators to reproduce. Some are directly toxic to the cell. In large numbers they might become overwhelming and life-threatening. We call them *infectious diseases*. The response needs to be correspondingly severe, and a more advanced system is activated.

Enter *the acquired immune system*. It includes a certain cell type called lymphocytes that produces antibodies or bullets. They measure the enemy to make projectiles that attach to it, put it in a choke hold, and kill it or spray it with more toxins. The only problem is that it takes a few days to fire up the factory. For this reason, they save the measurements and commit the patterns of the last intruder to memory in case of future attacks from a similar enemy. The factory is now programmed to produce the specific killer. Brilliant idea. We use this process of memorized attack substances as vaccines. We challenge the immune system with a microbe that has been rendered harmless to trigger the production of its own killing substance before the real thing shows up; this way we can respond without delay.

The two systems operate in steps, but make no mistake about it, they work as one. The bigger the threat, the more resources are put in motion. If the situation escalates, we may experience the full syndrome, including visible swelling and pain, a warning that things need fixing

Once the battle is won, a whole set of substances described earlier show up to end the inflammation and repair the damage. The battle may leave a messy field of pus and destruction. If the inflammation goes on long enough, there is replacement of destroyed cells with the formation of scar tissue. This is done by the inflammatory system as well. We now have an additional definition of illness: the battle between the attacker and the immune system.

We next consider *congenital or inborn genetic diseases*, where a single gene is expressing this disorder. They include conditions like inborn enzyme defects, malformations, Down syndrome, sickle cell anemia, cystic fibrosis, some forms of heart disease and some degenerative disorders. They tragically are less viable variants of our genome and fall at the low end of the bell curve we introduced earlier. Their numbers typically end up being around five percent. They are typically not inflammatory in nature. These are the situations where genetic therapies are the answer. Fortunately, we are beginning to see progress in this area of medicine.

Traumatic diseases have been considered self-explanatory, describing physically diagnoseable injuries, but this is no longer necessarily the case. For instance, new information has moved mental illnesses into a scenario where the trauma of mental stress can drive inflammation. Remember that all energy including thought energy may enter the signaling pathway and create a response; if the energy is negative enough, the response is inflammation. A well-known diagnosis is post-traumatic stress disorder (PTSD).

Simply put, trauma can lead to illness. This connection is called the social signal transduction theory of depression. It should ring a bell with us now that we are familiar with signal transduction and the nature of illness as a perturbance in our force field. These are examples of why disease classifications are becoming more confluent.

Chronic Inflammatory Illness—Most of Us Have One

This scenario explains the largest group of illnesses in our culture and also the least recognized: *chronic inflammatory disease.* Though we don't really understand the scope of this condition in all its forms, national statistics have some 2/3 of us overweight, and by implication harbingers of inflammatory disease.

It was first described as a cluster of disorders that showed up mainly in overweight patients. It was named syndrome X and went by the acronym of CHAOS, alluding to its components of high cholesterol, cardiovascular disease, adult onset diabetes, obesity and stroke. Because of its obvious manifestations, it was also called metabolic syndrome, inferring that there was something wrong with our metabolism.

To our surprise, we found that the underlying problem was not with our cells or metabolism; it is with what we do to it. Some of what we call food affects us negatively enough to make us sick. Heart disease and diabetes are major examples. We eventually came to understand that eating is one of the most important decisions we make on a daily basis. Edibles such as sugar and cholesterol may attach to cell walls and weaken the cell wall in the process. The immune system attacks and may end up destroying the underlying cells in a case of mistaken identity. In war this is collateral damage. Enlarged fat cells, cholesterol and fat are all immunotoxins.

Since these triggers are edibles from the energy metabolism, we could call the resulting illness metabolic. However, this is only one group of inflammatory agents.

Any candidate that does not support the body's life-affirming agenda is stopped at the door and may end up presented to the immune system as a toxin. It may be anything as toxic as asbestos or as insidious as pollen we breathe in or something we eat; or something we fail to do, like move. This probably comes as a surprise, but it is not a misprint. Sedentary lifestyle has been shown to be as damaging as smoking fifteen cigarettes a day!

We have now added another dimension to our definition of health. It is the seesaw relationship between our body's *thrive* and *defense*. If we think of all the possible challenges that knock on our cell doors every day, we understand that our homeland security has its hands full sorting this out.

What About Cancer?

It is well known that many chronic conditions carry increased cancer risk. If the attacker is too strong or the immune system itself is weakened, it is overwhelmed. We are learning of more and more cancers that start by festering for years as chronic low-grade inflammations. This might lead to constant cell destruction and repair.

The high cell turnover may lend itself to error while dividing and mutate into cancer cells. Remember the electronic flow of energy through the protein pathways that creates our health? This, in turn, can change genetic material or DNA, again leading to tissue changes called dysplasia metaplasia and neoplasia or malignancy. It has been shown that these pathways are interrupted in cancer. The same principle may be at work in autoimmune disease, allergies and other hypersensitivity reactions.

Once we understand the progression of the immune response, it makes sense that more and more types of cancer are shown to start with inflammation. If there were no immune system, we would succumb from minor invaders that would meet no resistance. This is the problem in immune-compromised persons. There is also a genetic link to genes in some cancer types, meaning we have to be extra vigilant with how we treat ourselves not to trigger those genes.

It might be more than coincidence that the list of cancer risks looks surprisingly like several risks for inflammatory disease: genetics, obesity, nutrition, alcohol and tobacco. In addition, we have a variety of other toxic chemicals in our environment that we don't even understand as carcinogens. We have a history of not recognizing triggers such as asbestos, lead, pesticides and benzene products. Toxic chemicals in general went under the radar for many years and taught us that if we don't look, we don't find.

Prolonged high stress might exhaust our resources and progress to irreversible stages. The definition of irreversible is not clearly defined and sometimes questioned, but one way to look at it will slowly emerge as we develop our thinking throughout this book.

The Immune System Has No Fear

Once called into action, the immune system does not quit, and this is a key point in chronic disease: immune cells fight blindly and have no fear. They die in numbers and replace themselves immediately and endlessly. Yet there are situations where the intruder is so strong and persistent that the system collapses. This is certainly true in the case of certain cancers.

Stress = Splinters

The common denominator of most acquired illnesses is the inflammatory reaction to an outside stressor or injury. Let's give it a big concrete metaphoric description that we can relate to: stress is splinters. From what we have learned so far about the mechanisms of illnesses, we can metaphorically redefine the stressors as a variety of splinters in our physical or mental finger that create negative current to incite inflammation and disturb the associated tissue and magnetic field.

We have no problem identifying bacilli and viruses as immune stressors. They can make us spectacularly ill and leave no doubt about their virulence. Neither would we try to defend ourselves against a lion by expecting our cells find a way to armor us against the lion's bite or demand our body find the strength to outrun the lion. While we would get a surge of adrenaline-induced strength, we reasonably recognize that the realistic choice is to act within our human boundaries. We would run, but the ultimate cure here would be to stop crossing paths with lions and stay out of their way. So then let us look at something curious: when it comes to those stressors we cannot see, our logic breaks down completely; we don't give much thought to what they are and how they affect us.

This can take on any form from thoughts to too much apple pie. Every time an inflammatory agent enters our body or brain, we are suffering a splinter, and the immune system has to try to get rid of it. If it does not, the hallmarks of inflammation may persist.

Doctor, What Do I Do About the Splinters?

What would you say if you went to a doctor who told you to keep the splinters and take medications to mask the pain of them being there? You could eventually get really sick. Hopefully, you would think this person incompetent and not follow this advice.

We hold ourselves to be reasonable, intelligent beings, and so we would not keep splinters and walk around as vats of inflammation chomping on pills to keep it silent. Yet this is precisely what we are doing in treating chronic conditions with remedies to silence the symptoms. We know this is true because we slowly get worse over time, needing stronger and stronger remedies to keep the developing reaction in check. And we slowly feel worse and worse. In quantum language we fail to see the whole and are more concerned with content than process.

Let us replay this whole scenario. You see the doctor for diabetes caused by nutrition, or respiratory illness caused by toxic air. Either splinter will shorten your life, possibly disable you before you die.

What Should the Doctor Tell You?
And What Will You Do?

This is a pointed scenario and a pointed question lest you should miss the point: if we look at what we have discussed so far, health emerges as a relationship between the body and its environment. Illness is the battleground between the offending agent and the immune system; wellness being when the immune system is shut off and stays off. We already have a core definition of good health: the absence of immunologic stress and the presence of positive reinforcement. Treatment starts with removal of the splinter!

Research bears this out in all areas of our lives. We can show the positive energy or health benefits of anything from positive encouragement to eating our vegetables. Now that we can contemplate illness from an energy standpoint, it opens the door to healing by resetting our magnetic state. As long as the splinter remains, it is kind of like Lucy in the chocolate factory; it will reinforce the injury current faster than we can reset it.

Our Lifestyle Illnesses: Lack of Medications

It almost looks absurd on paper, but when you think about it, this is a prevailing view of health care today. If you are sick, it is for lack of medications. Or because you are not taking the right medicine! You are barraged with the idea that your body needs some medication to be healthy. Feeling down? Can't sleep? High cholesterol or blood sugar? Whatever the reason, you need a pill, a remedy to make it go away, to feel up, to calm down, to deal with life.

Once we have defined health as taking several pills to get through a day, we depend on symptom-masking "life-style medications". The pharmaceutical industry drives this dependency by funding research that invents new diagnoses and lowers guidelines for prescribing medication. For instance, it is true that it is better to have lower blood pressure. High blood pressure may be only one of the many manifestations of inflammation. Overweight by itself is a risk because enlarged fat cells are inflammatory. We patch that one up, and the proteome has other pathways to express it: high blood sugar, high cholesterol, gastritis, arthritis and so on. If we are generally overweight and unhealthy, driving our blood pressure below ever-lower guidelines is not going to take us out of the risk category that our weight puts us in.

On the other hand, healthy persons who follow these guidelines may be convinced to take medications they don't really need, thus becoming patients, and also experience so-called side effects of the medications.

Whatever the reasons for ingesting chemicals unknown to the body, remember, they interface with the proteome governed by quantum laws of probabilities and uncertainty, and may have unpredictable effects.

Medicine has inadvertently given us the largest, most vivid illustration of this by administering chemicals and other forms of energy with unknown travel paths through the proteome. The predictably unpredictable results are called side effects.

They Are Effects

These are not side effects; they are effects on a quantum system of an unknown substance. If you look at late night TV where the injury lawyers advertise their business, you know that medications may cause anything from weakness, brain fog, stroke and depression to loss of limb or life. People who take medications often do not even realize how reduced they are before they try to keep up with a well person.

Despite clinical trials, the full effect on different individuals of medications becomes a guessing game, as I am sure you have noticed. Yet when you turn on your TV, you are bombarded by images of glamorous, happy patients taking drug X, Z and Y and living in picture-perfect harmony with each other and nature. The next thing you know is a big ad on TV urging you to call a law firm if someone you know took such-and such a drug and lost a limb, or you lost a relative to this drug—the drug of bucolic idyll.

One could say that taking medications would be like fixing a piece of jewelry with a sledgehammer. They might hit anywhere, even destroy the piece, because it is uncertain where its power might strike. You can now begin to see the tunnel vision and also the danger in accepting medications as panaceas.

Death by Prescription

"Taking prescribed medications is the fourth leading cause of death among Americans," per staff writer Michael Schroeder in *U.S. World & News Report* in 2016. That translated into some one hundred thousand individuals.

Despite all this, we let ourselves be told that we can keep the splinter and instead take potions to overcome it! They peddle the Kool-Aid, and we gladly drink it. Such is the business of medicine and pharmacology. Meanwhile, our slowly aching, breaking bodies tell us differently.

We get what we ask for. The majority of inflammatory illness is self-inflicted. Statistics show that the majority of us will visit a doctor and be diagnosed with some metabolic derangement necessitating medications by the latest community standards of medical care. In fact, we might even be told we have some syndrome invented by the drug industry.

After exhausting the cholesterol and sugar-related market, they were looking to expand. This led to the promulgation of bogus or unrecognized mental-health diagnoses in the 1990's.

Treating the Nuisance

All of a sudden new mental-health diagnoses, especially in unruly children, started cropping up. A favorite is ODD. The full medical terminology is Intermittent Oppositional Defiant Disorder, otherwise known as Occasionally Being a Nuisance. You might recognize this syndrome from your own life. Both my husband and I have suffered bouts of this condition in our thirty years of marriage.

I ran across a stubborn case of ODD in my wanderings in the backwoods of California. A mother told me she took her ill-behaved young son to a "crystal therapist," where rock crystals are pressed against the body to drive out unbearable behavior. "It worked," she beamed. "In addition, we started being nicer to him, and he was cured!" Not to negate crystal therapy. However, she might have done well, possibly even saved the rock therapy, if she had read a book by the Swiss child psychiatrist, Alice Miller, called *The Drama of the Gifted Child*. But it seems she did remove the splinter.

I have been invited to medical seminars touting sleeplessness as a dire, most treatable problem. Every person goes through periods of sleeplessness, especially in periods of stress or worry, and might need help problem-solving instead of becoming addicted to sleeping pills. The biggest heist by the drug industry was when it cornered the pain market with the mantra that pain was a neglected condition. Opioid painkillers were let loose to create our worst public-health epidemic since the rise of sugar-related disease. We are still at a loss to solve it and all the other conditions we create and wring our hands over.

The Real Issue

This should come as no surprise by now: the real issue is a sea-shift in our economic and political systems including public health. Unfortunately, there is no meaningful voice or lobby for wellness while the financial stakes for the drug industry are enormous and their lobby watertight.

If this sounds like I am some fanatic antimedicine "naturalist," I am not. Being a medical doctor, I am rooted in orthodox medicine.

We need to push the frontiers, but we have failed to start out by grounding ourselves in the basic knowledge of the processes that govern our health.

Only a small number of us should be ill enough to risk these interventions, and we should not be made into "medical customers". We should train our doctors to understand wellness as much as we do illness.

The amazing thing is that if we removed the triggers, there would be a 75 percent reduction in patients and the stuff they consume. For the US being the greatest country on earth, we are amazingly small-minded and pessimistic. We think our economy will go under if we go positive and accept modern science, stop eating sugar, opioids and vaping materials, burning oil and selling weapons. And this is the land of positive-thinking? It is said that you cannot teach a man anything new if his livelihood depends on the old. It is so sad that we cannot see enough opportunities in getting rid of our splinters while building up a thriving society. Instead we are the culture of duped consumers and quick fixes. The old travelling-medicine show is only a step away. We buy more self-help books than any other nation, and yet we are fatter, sicker and more addicted.

We tacitly accept that life is a process of ailing and weakening, and our prospects grow bleaker by the decade. This is confirmed by our longevity statistics; they are stagnating, in fact, going down. Our reality is, instead of healing ourselves, we call on illness and keep calling.

Instead of information and support, there is a candy stand at the checkout counter. My local hospital purports to promote health, but the subliminal message is a "Sweet Treat Bakery" in the lobby. We have worldwide problems. According to UN statistics, 9 out of 10 people are victims of polluted air, "the new tobacco".

It is a sad statement about us that we have let it come to this. As with our other follies, this ignorance is not an excuse. The environment charges us with the responsibility for sorting out what is good for us, and we get what we ask for.

We Need to Know

We do understand that if we buy a shiny new car, we need to maintain it. You get the point: we neglect and treat our body worse than a replaceable car. We have no maintenance plan and give no thought to the fact that we only get one. We even delude ourselves into thinking there will be replacement parts readily available because science will figure something out. Tell that to transplant recipients who have met their HLA receptors. Let us remind ourselves again: no scientist has ever repaired a cell, but the cell does not need repair. It needs to be bathed in positive energy.

Surely you now realize that health is not something we bring home in a pill box from the doctor's office. Nor is it a fit of "dieting" while holding our breath to fit into a dress for an occasion. It is the sum of what we take down from the universe over our lifetime.

You also understand that in this context, all input such as thoughts, waves, and matter is information that triggers our genes to write the story of our health.

So what is the information that, combined with our given genetic potential, will write the story of our health and well being? We can think of it in groups forming four pieces of the health pie. Since they all can make it or break it for us, we'll look at them separately. They are

1. what we eat,
2. how we move,
3. what we think,
4. where we live.

CHAPTER 3
What We Eat

Our Eating Makes All the Difference

Nutrition is a misunderstood and neglected area of medicine. The truth is, we lack meaningful training because we cannot agree on the science involved. This is a regrettable abdication of responsibility for one of the main causes of illness. Being a medical doctor and nutritionist myself, I had not understood how critical it is to our health, how little we understand of it and how distorted and confusing it is until I saw patients changing their nutrition get well from chronic illnesses, reconnect with old dreams and create new lives for themselves.

It was a most humbling experience, but also a most rewarding one, because its importance sank in with me. I started digging in the literature and found more than I bargained for. I wrote a book explaining how the body and nutrition work together to create our weight and health. It became my platform for thinking through the other origins of illnesses. It also drove me to the typewriter to share this with as many people as possible.

A Fateful Relationship

We know our nutrition is not working for us because we are currently experiencing abysmal results of unhealthy eating. Obesity, ill health, psychiatric problems, low quality of life and premature death are bankrupting our health budget. As we will see, nutrition influences all our behavior, including how well we learn. Close to

20 percent of our GNP is spent on health care, mostly on chronic illnesses with paltry results.

Some 40 percent of Medicare is spent on diabetes, and no one is getting better, just slowly worse.

Yet we seem to discount the facts and ignore the gravity of the burden this places on us.

Perhaps understanding the situation in its realistic detail will bring it closer to home and into the realm of things we both can and need to change.

The Malnutrition of the Rich

Eating in famine and in surplus are equally problematic. In famine one gleans what it takes to stay alive, though not healthy. We see pictures of half-starved people lacking protein and calories. In our culture, the issue is that we have a surplus of edibles, but not all edibles are foods. It would be more to the point to say that there is a surplus of potential splinters posing as food, and we don't grasp this. We, the overfed and overweight of the land of plenty, might not look like the starving, but we suffer the malnutrition of the rich.

What is Good Nutrition?

The object of the body is to turn food stuffs into electrical power and not splinters. To relate to this, we have to look at the process itself. If not, we end up in the philosophy department.

Most "experts" seem to operate in that realm. I hear a lot of interesting statements about nutrition at parties. "The reason s/he is overweight is that s/he has a food allergy." "Artificial sweeteners cause seizures." "Red meat causes cancer." None of these statements are backed by science, but they are passed around like gospel.

Admittedly, nutritional research is difficult to carry out because we cannot lock people up long term and feed them selectively. In population studies we oftentimes have to rely on self-reporting. If you have ever taken a nutritional history from anyone, you know that this is close to useless.

My patients who gained four pounds on "eating lettuce" wanted to be agreeable and oftentimes told me what they thought I wanted to hear. They also were in serious denial, hard pressed to remember the cake and candy that followed the lettuce. The kind of time and soul-searching it took to get a real history is not really feasible in the primary care setting. Meanwhile, if good information finds its way to the patient, not to mention if the patient abides by it, the body responds very quickly to good nutrition. Medicine claims to be "evidence based," but finds it hard to accept this time-proven evidence.

What Is Good Food?

Some simple food chemistry: We draw our calories from 3 groups of food groups: Protein, fat and carbohydrates. Oh, there is alcohol, but it is not defined as a food.

Protein contains nitrogen, which is indispensable to animal life. Its source is mainly animal products. We have seen how our lean working body is a network of structural and messenger proteins. These are constantly turned over or used for repair and so a reliable supply is basic to good health. Our basic protein requirements are still the subject of much turbulence, though it has been known and described over and over in the literature. A rule of thumb is one gram of protein per kilo of normal body weight per day.

The standard established by the National Task Force for the Prevention and Treatment of Obesity in 1993 comes in a tad lower at .8 gram per kilo with allowances for stress like weight loss and pregnancy. When Dr. Atkins got on the right track, denouncing sugar and promoting protein, he was dragged in front of a bribed, ill-informed Congress and almost defrocked. Since then, protein has been more or less "dangerous" for bizarre and unscientific reasons. It is almost as though we fear the truth. I know of no person who killed him/herself eating protein, but I know of millions committing slow suicide by sugar.

Fat is our storage and insulation material. It is a main ingredient in cell walls and certain hormones. The composition of human fat is some 45 percent unsaturated, 45 percent saturated and 10 percent essential fats of omega-3 and 6 types. The brain is somewhat different, including more omega-3, which acts as an anti-inflammatory agent all through the body. Essential simply means that the body cannot produce this precious substance; it has to be ingested. We need these fats, though in small daily amounts. Our sources are both from animals and plants. We have correctly identified fish oil as a main source of omega-3.

There is another aspect of food: it might influence the strength of our battery. While we have several strong pH buffer systems, it might not be a fluke that a balanced meal supplies acid through meat and dairy, but plant-based foods are alkaline.

We see again that nature thrives on balance between elements.

In Sheep's Clothing

If sugar powers our batteries, it seems like a good thing, right? Unfortunately, here is another of life's many lessons.

Let us start by writing the sequence of energy production:

Sugar→chemical energy (ATP)→electric power across the cell membrane (battery)→cells use this voltage potential to run the body.

If we heeded this and ate to power our cells, that would be the end of this chapter. Think about it.

The problem comes when we eat excess refined sugars, because they are not used in the energy production. They leave this flow and start wandering. To get a handle on this, we need to understand how sugar processed by the body.

Sugar is the nutritional wild card, the large group known as carbohydrates. All plants are carbohydrates consisting of varying degrees of sugar and fiber. The more fiber, the less sugar and vice versa. The power or intensity of a sugar is gauged on a scale called the Glycemic Index, arbitrarily ranging from 0 for fiber to 100 for the strongest or most refined sugar, expressing the ability of a sugar to trigger the production of insulin in our pancreas. Insulin carries sugar into the cells. The more refined the sugar, meaning the higher the GI, the more insulin is needed. Though biochemical texts make this point, the consequences of this relationship are not well understood.

Setting the Sugar-Insulin Thermostat

Sugar and insulin run a thermostat for our weight and health that functions as follows:

When we eat a balanced, healthy meal of protein, fat and complex sugars from vegetables, legumes and fruits, sugar is carried slowly into the cells and burned, keeping the blood sugar normal.

Sugar and insulin oscillate gently up and down within a window of normal values; our body stays normal weight, and our metabolism is set for good health. On the other hand, if we take in large amounts of refined sugar, our pancreas responds very fast by pouring out high amounts of insulin, or the sugar will pile up in our bloodstream. One would think more is better, but aye, there is a rub.

The excess has to go somewhere. It is turned into fat and cholesterol, and we gain weight. That means our weight thermostat goes up. Insulin overshoots, our blood sugar plummets, and we become hypoglycemic.

At the new low, we now need more quick sugar to pick us up. We start seeing large blood sugar swings, too high or too low, and our energy and mood follow. If we keep eating sugar, the cell will literally start closing the door, meaning, "Thank you, but I am full." If we don't listen and continue overeating, sugar, fat and insulin pile up both in the cell and in the bloodstream, and we have trouble.

Insulin Resistance

The first phase of this development is high sugar needing high insulin to truck it into the cell. We produce more insulin, our blood sugar still registers as normal; but all is not well because high insulin is by itself inflammatory, and our "normal blood sugar" begins to back up to "high normal." This is pathology in the making; a favorite child with many names: hyperinsulinemia, insulin resistance or pre-diabetes. If we continue piling up the sugar, we raise our risk for chronic illness culminating in diabetes. Since we don't measure insulin, this first sign is not registered, and the subsequent ones are treated with medications.

If we think back on our new-found understanding of the cell, recall that sugar is the raw material for our electric energy.

However, *excess* blood sugar, fat and insulin all become runaway and show up as triggers of the transduction pathways, activating the immune system, which in turn attacks fat cells and other structures. If the pH, electrolyte or electrical system are compromised, these effects become more pronounced.

This is how sugar-related inflammation happens. It hits the body where we have genetic predispositions to disorders like diabetes, hypertension, cardiovascular disease and other inflammatory illnesses. In short, we see that we have a self-perpetuating loop of weight gain and inflammatory illness based on high sugar.

Here is the cycle of events that describes how insulin resistance happens:

high sugar→insulin→fat/cholesterol→weight→activation of the immune system→inflammation→illness→sugar.

It is an open cascading system where each step can multiply and intensify their effects.

Sugar, the Splinter

And here are some key points: only high sugar can trigger high insulin, and only insulin can turn sugar to fat. As we pointed out earlier, the body does not really need sugar since it can convert fat and protein to sugar-like links in energy production process. Also, the overproduction of sugar and insulin is a stress response that raises blood sugar further.

High sugar spawns fat and cholesterol. The latter two are blamed in cardiovascular disease, but as we see, they have the same mother. While the chain usually starts with sugar, we can also enter the chain at the point of fat cells (or weight gain) by eating fat, but most people do not drink oil or eat lard, and their fat production comes largely from eating sugar.

This loop links the energy production pathway with that of transduction. It explains how sugar, insulin, weight and inflammatory illnesses are linked.

2/3 of Us Are Unhealthy

It is a staggering estimate, but some 2/3 of all Americans are overweight, implying insulin resistance. Though most chronic illness happens within this context, it is not recognized until the blood sugar rises to our defined abnormal. By this time, insulin has already been high for a long time, and inflammatory diseases may already have developed.

Since high insulin is not seen as a matter of urgency, we don't test for it. In fact, testing is a waste of time as long as we don't lower it but only treat symptoms, especially since the treatment actually raises insulin instead of lowering it. You read it right. This is what we do when we take medications instead of reversing the process right here by lowering the sugar intake to curb insulin production. Would the latter work? Yes, and the proof is in the pudding, eh, the patient. Sugar-free, of course.

The list of inflammatory diseases is growing, and not without reason. An alphabetical list of diagnoses from the literature includes Alzheimer's, ankylosing spondylitis, arthritis (osteoarthritis, rheumatoid arthritis [RA], psoriatic arthritis), asthma, atherosclerosis, Crohn's disease, colitis, dermatitis, diverticulitis, fibromyalgia, hepatitis, irritable bowel syndrome (IBS), systemic lupus erythematous (SLE), nephritis, Parkinson's disease and ulcerative colitis. This is only a sampling. At this point, it might be more pertinent to ask which chronic diseases are not inflammatory.

Diabetes

When the sugar load becomes so high that our insulin production collapses, we get chronic high blood sugar known as diabetes. Antidiabetic medications squeeze the exhausted pancreas to produce more insulin. While lowering blood sugar, it increases its poisonous effects. It is tantamount to beating the perennial dead horse. Has this ever been explained to a diabetic patient, I wonder.

Whatever the point of entry into the cycle, the common final result is inflammation. Remember the immune response includes increased stress hormones. They also raise blood sugar, meaning illness itself raises blood sugar, closing the vicious cycle into a loop. We have just seen that sugar is not a food. It is the original mother splinter.

Diabetes type 2 is the prototype of full-blown sugar-poisoning syndrome. The effects are staggering: high levels of sugar, breakdown products of sugar, insulin and breakdown products of insulin are all toxic and worsen inflammation. They all circulate and seed complications throughout the body. It is more insidious and harmful than we realize, because slow sugar-poisoning contributes to physical and mental disability. It is a chronic low-grade generalized inflammation that attacks large and small blood vessels, causing cardiovascular disease, reduced circulation to the legs and damage to organs like kidneys and eyes. It can cause widespread and debilitating neurological problems including brain atrophy, slow mentation, depression, slow walking, fatigue and sleep disturbances.

Diabetes type 2 is also a prototype of a reversible poisoning condition. It responds willingly to stopping sugar.

Yet I hear repeatedly, "I have diabetes type 2, but they gave me medicine for it." The patient is lulled into thinking that s/he is "treated." No information, no alternative. No public health effort. The medications used to treat chronic diseases such as diabetes type 2 crop up with regular intervals on TV in infomercials for injury lawyers who make a living chasing life-and-limb-threatening effects of these medications. You already know that they are wild cards in the proteome.

While eating is not the only source of inflammation, we could call the nutritional variety what it really is: sugar eater's syndrome or sugar-poisoning.

Another Look at Insulin, the Determinator

Insulin is much more than the switch of our sugar metabolism. It is the master switch that needs to be on for all the other switches to work. This makes it our main anabolic hormone, meaning it governs the building up of living tissues from the nutritional elements of amino acids and fatty acids. It also regulates the production of eicosanoids, making it part of immune regulation. It helps regulate electrolyte excretion by the kidneys. This brings our thoughts to energy metabolisms.

High insulin causes water retention in the body that goes away almost instantly by lowering insulin. Polycystic ovarian syndrome responds to lowering insulin by promoting pregnancy. Brain function is maximal at normal insulin. Aside from dietary intake, our body can produce cholesterol from what we call activated sugar. Its metabolism is ultimately run by insulin, as is the synthesis of hormones and enzymes, which is another way of saying that if insulin is out of the normal window, we are at risk for any malfunction in any of our body's metabolic systems. Remember the inflammatory loop. All this while your blood sugar might be read as normal; and so, the question is always the same: what raised your insulin?

Foods Becomes Poison along the Sliding Scale

It cannot be said often enough; the answer to the above question is always the same: sugar. This begs the next question: if you eat something that makes you ill, would that be a food? Again, your brain knows the answer, but that might not count for much, so let us be reasonable. It would be a poison. This should be our warning to stop thinking a calorie is a calorie. What calories you eat make all the difference. Complicating the matter is that the transition between the food and potential poison is a sliding one.

The Sliding Scale

The GI scale of sugars starts on the low end with vegetables, legumes, lower than 40. Fruit falls in the middle (GI around 50) and is good in small doses but can raise blood sugar if eaten in large quantities. Edibles with GI higher than 50 start out as foods but become toxins if overeaten. We know that an apple a day etc., but a pound of apples a day would represent too much fruit sugar.

At high GI, sugars become dangerous (grains and table sugar are in the GI range of 70 and over). By the way, beer is off the GI scale at 105. If you are in doubt, there is an easy way to tell where a sugar falls on the GI scale. Ask yourself if it is strong enough to ferment into alcohol. Fruit makes wine (medium strength) while grains and potatoes make pure liquors (high strength). The GI of vegetables is too low to support fermentation, thus too low to derail to your sugar-insulin thermostat, while the natural sugars in grasses and trees are so tightly bound only animals have the enzymes to digest them.

If we keep a low GI diet to set our fasting blood sugar at about 80mg/dl and fasting insulin levels around 6mIU/L or less, we have effectively removed sugar-related health risk. The corresponding long-term blood sugar would be (HbA1c) of 5.5% or less. This means that our average meal should be no more than GI 40 or so. There is a plethora of studies in the literature to confirm this. Inflammation can be created in one meal and stopped over a short time of good eating. The takeaway here again is the same: strong sugars/grains are not food groups; they are potentially toxic additives and best used that way. It should be said that very coarsely milled grains yield high fiber, lowering GI. Unfortunately they are considered "gritty" and routinely refined to high GI level.

What inflammatory illnesses we get from eating sugar depends on our genetic predisposition. For instance, my family history includes a raft of diabetes type 2. I, therefore, by definition, have abnormal sugar metabolism. All I have to do to become diabetic is to eat sugar and become overweight. I do understand that I have this tendency, but my genes will serve me well if I respect this knowledge. I have a choice to live disease-free. Considering the toll chronic illness takes on us individually and as a society, it seems to me we should help each other to live better instead of dreaming about remedies to mask whatever manifestations of the poor choices we make.

How Is Your Nutrition?

Now that we have decided that food is found at low GI, things become very interesting. Right off the bat we have eliminated most of what we eat: cereal for breakfast, hamburger for lunch and pizza for dinner. We stand little chance of normal insulin and a resting immune system on this eating program.

Lack of protein is called wasting disease. So what is lack of sugar called? Good health, that is what. A relative lack is optimal, meaning lack of refined, but access to complex ones. We have the luxury of living in colors, those of fruits and vegetables that give us fiber, polyphenols or antioxidants and other immune-strengthening compounds. They are not essential to life, but are a lush addition to make our diet complete. This sums up the paleo-type eating, which is how we ate when our metabolism evolved. Another thing to understand is the designation "essential." There are essential amino acids and essential fats, meaning they cannot be produced by the body, but have to be eaten. Are there any essential carbohydrates or sugars? Enough said.

I am appalled at the amount of misinformation and confusion I see out there. There is an urgent need to inform ourselves and our children on the basics of nutrition outlined here. If you would like to see a graphic representation of the blood-sugar curve and how to eat low GI to set your blood sugar, you will find it in my book on nutrition.

But there is more to know before we can maneuver our way through the nutrition labyrinth.

Our Hunger Thermostats

The ultimate thermostat of hunger and eating rests, not surprisingly, with the CEO, the brain, because it makes the final decisions on most of what we do in life. It can be set independent of eating. Remember the appetite suppressant medications that were all the rage some twenty years ago? They simply shut off the brain thermostat. The downside here was that the brain read "full" while the body was starving. As soon as this effect wore off, the body claimed back all the missing calories and then some.

The brain thermostat can also be manipulated by brain surgery, though this has never proven a popular weight-control method. In addition, we also have a thermostat that responds to volume. When we overeat to stretch the stomach, we need to eat more and more to become full. All these ways of raising our thermostats lead to the same thing: high blood sugar, high insulin, weight gain and inflammation. Raising insulin is kind of like letting the cat out of the box.

Sugar Is Physically Addictive

It gets worse. Sugar is not just toxic; it is also very addictive, physically and psychologically. If you read opinions on the internet, you will see how we think about sugar: "The food nobody needs but everybody craves," or "Sugar drives behavioral responses consistent with addiction." Hello? Refined sugar is not a food. It does not drive "addiction-like behaviors." It *is* addictive, if not by decree of medicine then at least by dictionary definition and by action on the brain. I am not sure what else is needed to understand this. For the record, addiction is defined by most dictionaries as "repeated involvement in a substance or activity that may be harmful, but is continued because it causes pleasure." Recognize anything?

The physically addictive properties of sugar are explained by the large swings in the blood sugar and insulin curve when taken in high doses. Our blood sugar is either high or low but never settles at normal. This is a physical addiction curve driven by low blood sugar and can cause mood swings, depression and anxiety. It becomes a slalom curve between euphoric fullness and the fatigue of low blood sugar. The only way off this curve is to remove the sugar and eat slow metabolizing, filling foods, including protein and fiber to lower the curve out of the inflammatory range.

Double Whammy: Sugar Is Also Psychologically Addictive

We are complicated creatures, and so it is with our nutrition. Equipped with our capacity for emotions, we tie most of what we do to how we feel about things. Our brain is sometimes tricked into making decisions that are not necessarily good for us.

It has been shown that sugar works over the brain receptors of dopamine and enkephalins in an area of the brain called the pleasure center. Some call this area the reptilian brain because it evades reason. It has been a long haul, but sugar has finally been shown to use the same neural pathways in the brain as do other addictive drugs. Overdosing on sugar thus elicits the same response. This is a reward system tied to powerful forces such as euphoria, love and motivation. We could get used to that, and we do.

The psychological addictive properties come with our complex behavior around sugar. We might have grown up in a cultural setting where sugar was used as reward/comfort. We were lovingly given a cookie if we cried. Or we were stuffing holes in our souls, so to speak, with sugar. Whether we are mad, glad, or sad, too many of us have learned to tie eating sweets to feeling better. We are not talking tofu here; we are specifically referring to edibles that give us the "sugar high." Many understand this principle and freely declare, "I am a sugar addict," without giving much thought to what addiction really means.

We Are Addicted to Illness

Our sugar addiction is truly the other opioid epidemic of our time in terms of cost to society. We spend our lives as patients and get used to decreasing quality of life with increasing limitations and debilitation. We need chronic medical care while we decry the bills attached to it. We stagger around like Frankenstein's creations held together by sugar and medications. While we cast aspersions on alcohol addicts, we find this addiction almost cute. The lack of logic is screaming at us again: if we declared ourselves addicted to alcohol or refused to wear seat belts, both of which maim and kill less than overdosing on sugar, it certainly would not be considered cute.

Addictions Can Be Epigenetic

Recall the regulators of genes called epi-genes. They are triggered by the environment and can change us without changing our genes. These changes may be passed on to the next generations. Thus, a predisposition for obesity, diabetes and other diseases can be passed on without our genes changing. In short, these addictions are not dictated by our genes; they are dictated to our genes by our behavior. So much for the dogma that genes decide our fate.

A Case of Mistaken Identity

Meanwhile, China has become the dubious diabetic chart topper. According to Jeff Kingston, director of Asian studies at Temple University, Japan, "Asia is on track to become the global epicenter for diabetes as dietary habits change and people become less active. Currently there are about 138 million diabetics in Asia, and this is projected to rise to 215 million by 2040." So much for the skinny noodle eaters.

We are dominated by a gigantic food and pharmaco-medical industry that started getting out of hand in the 1960s. It has managed to thwart research into blaming fat instead of sugar for obesity ever since, pushing of everything from cholesterol medications to surgery, catering to our ignorance and addiction.

The Great Squabble

With the inflammatory epidemic, the great squabble began. We could not agree on what caused the problem or how to solve it. Philosophers, scientists, gurus, prophets, film stars, politicians, even doctors became authorities on diets and sought to corner the nutrition market. This led to the endless and useless discussion with less scientific and more political elements at work. It also led to the food pyramid of 1993, and the problem exploded into the situation we see today.

We already then had the biochemical information to explain what healthy nutrition looks like. Still we keep up the squabble while we watch ourselves grow unhealthier, not only in the US but all around the globe.

When sugar finally was spotlighted, there was the ludicrous diversion of the issue by inventing the evils of cornstarch and the bogeyman soft drinks. What you were not told was that if you cannot have your fix from a can, you will find it from a cookie.

The chairman of the nutrition department of a prestigious university in my neighborhood was scandalized when I suggested we can live without sugar. He beseeched upon me to consider the need for it to maintain blood sugar. He probably never heard about our Alaskan neighbors, the Inuit, who lived without carbohydrates and also without cardiovascular disease or diabetes for thousands of years before they met up with our lifestyle.

The Inuit diet narrowed it down to the essentials for life sustenance: protein and mostly marine fats. It turns out to be these two and not much else. Lacking bulk, they might have suffered constipation and lifespan was low, as could be expected in the foreboding arctic climate. They ran no homes for the aged. But as a culture they lived practically carbohydrate-free. Vitamins are micronutrients essential to the functioning of body processes. As was proven by those same Eskimos, those can be gleaned through raw meat and fat.

I never met a patient who got fat from eating protein or fat. Sugar was always the problem. Fat is self-limiting. You can only eat so much before you don't want any more. When I specifically asked about the fats eaten, it always came down to the crackers, chips, bread and fast food, all of which are largely sugars. No one gave me a history of eating lard or drinking oil. On the other hand, when fat is mixed with sugar, it helps raise the thermostat; we eat more and the calories from the fat are stored even faster. That is why the dessert comes last, there is always room for it.

The most recent calamity for our health was the aforementioned food pyramid of 1993. It was tantamount to a freefall into the sugar bowl. Created by people with more authority than knowledge of the subject, it plunged society into the depth of sugar addiction we are seeing now.

Of all the patients who came to me, including a number of health professionals, almost no one understood this. Our lack of education and information still leaves us helpless to do anything about it.

Information can be conveyed to persons of any age and should be part of any school or training curriculum. If we all understood the same thing, it would be much easier to cooperate around good health. This would involve a massive public-health outreach and policy changes. We could make informed decisions and reinforce positive behavior as a society to promote good health instead of bad.

I have taught nutrition to thousands of people from all walks of life including health personnel and lectured to groups of all sizes. Sadly, most of them are caught in the addiction cycle. It would have been so much better had they never become addicted. Still I am encouraged because on average, one in twenty of my listeners reports back to me that this information reached them and changed their lives. That is 5 percent from a single lecture. I also saw health miracles in my office patients.

The problem was long-term maintenance because they went back into the environment that created them, and there was little or no support. In fact, the opposite would sometimes be the case. Patients told me stories about friends bringing them homemade cookies and other sweet treats and telling them to "worry about their weight some other time." We advise alcoholic patients not to keep the company of their comrades at the bar, but there is no sugar-free environment unless we dream ourselves back to Japan some years ago when brined salmon was a high-end breakfast. This tells us that we have to create the context in which constructive habits can thrive, a context where good eating is prized and valued. How long, Lord, how long before we act?

Food Is Not Addictive

From the vantage point of nutrition, we can now define health as an ongoing tug-of-war between food and sugar to set our insulin thermostat. When first refined, sugar was actually thought a drug and sold for unspecified medicinal purposes. Its addictive properties are still sailing under the radar, making it one of the most insidious and dangerous ones we take daily. So how do we eat "drug-free"?

Let us repeat the basic lesson of defining the ingredients that keep the thermostat on low: protein, vegetables, legumes, fruits and small amounts of fat. Second lesson: remember the structure and function of the cell; enough protein to support the cell itself and its network that runs our energy flow. Protein keeps insulin low and can be turned into building blocks or be burned as sugar. Third lesson: we are in the lucky situation of having a rainbow of colored fruits and vegetables available to add bulk and strength. A small amount of good oil rounds out this paleo-type program. Eating this way shuts off the hunger thermostat, allowing the body to produce energy without risking excess sugar activating the immune system.

My patients used this type of program and saw their health change in short order. I spent months and years surveilling the medical literature to back up my clinical observations with mainstream research. I then wrote a book on nutrition "The Food Tree" to explain what we need to do with respect to food to recover our health.

I was dismissed as irrelevant and probably a bit daft when in 2010 I presented this information to four hundred physicians. Everyone over fifty years old left the room in silence while the junior contingency was obviously curious and wanted to know more. No discussion followed, only silent condemnation. I can only imagine what the same crew of experts would think of this book. Since this is how our so-called leaders think, it's not easy to find answers.

How Does Addiction happen?

How do we explain the appearance of epidemics of addiction? They came on over a time span far too short to be explained by our genetic makeup. Now let us think back at the bell curve where we saw distributions of traits in a normal population.

Since addiction is not passed on by single gene inheritance, its numbers in a population would be predictable on that sort of curve. A few of us would be very susceptible, a few not at all and most of us in the middle would be susceptible if the addictive agent were foisted on us. Addictive substances have one thing in common: before their mass production and mass marketing, there was no crisis. Their easy availability and the deliberate aggressive promotion of their use have shifted the curve to create the addictive epidemics we are seeing now.

This is what happened with alcohol. It eventually led to prohibition. We had the cigarette scourge, not to mention the current opioid and vaping disaster. The more exposure, the more users, since these poisons are labelled as "helpful" or "treats." The point is, addiction epidemics come because they are labelled desirable parts of our lifestyle. Conversely, they go away when we recognize their damage and institute education and policy interventions to stop them.

Addiction is better prevented than treated.

Whether to opioids or sugar, addiction is not to be trifled with because the recovery rate of its victims is abysmal. Those who take up the challenge are in an uphill battle. Weight losers and other addicts clean up, get healthier, only to "crack" and regain all their weight, health problems and then some. The permanent recovery rate from any addiction is variable but low. To our credit, we have conquered other health scourges. However, it takes time, and the impetus to do it typically does not come from our leaders. It comes from the grassroot.

So why don't we hear from the grassroot? Because we are sugar-addicted as a culture. Where are the "mothers against sugar"? There is silence because we, the mothers, are addicted and powerless to help ourselves or our children. We strive to give them a nice life and send them to good schools, but we are blithely destroying their health. Research has shown budding arteriosclerotic disease in arteries of ten-year-olds, and adolescents are now hospitalized for adult onset diabetes.

In 2003, the World Health Organization made an attempt to campaign for a worldwide 10 percent reduction in sugar consumption. The American sugar lobby nixed it, and that was the end of it. Meanwhile, there is sugar in almost everything we buy, from soup to salad, and the cost to society is untold.

"But we have to eat" is an argument I often hear. This is not a serious argument; it is simply ignorance speaking. One could also say, "But we have to drink." We don't need to drink alcohol or poison to quench our thirst any more than we need to eat sugar and make ourselves ill to settle hunger.

Maybe we need a little bit of the pasta diet: we walk pasta bakery, we walk pasta candy store, pasta ice-cream store. Let's make this simple: we walk pasta everything that raises our insulin. Let us celebrate that we can revel in the luxury of the fresh produce aisle and the fact that we have all this abundance available to us.

Lifestyle Drugs: The Silver Bullets

We are the culture of self-helpers. Millions of books to lose weight and gain health have been written by duchesses and magicians; health gurus have come and gone. We have lived through the miracles of grapefruit, melon rind, green coffee beans, various teas, even vinegar. Then there is juicing. It, of course, destroys the fiber in food, indeed landing us in the fountain of youth, since we are now eating baby food. Resveratrol was a big one for the heart that got us sipping wine. Alas, it waned too.

When you hear nonsense such as tomato paste being defined as a serving of vegetables, you are right to wonder. At one moment our great hope is attached to celery, making this pedestrian green stalk almost a black-market item for a couple of months till the disillusionment sets in and the next fifteen-minute wonder crops up. We have a billion-dollar industry selling hope, silver bullets and overnight miracles. Once they don't work, we graduate to the medico-pharma industry. Stronger drugs have ever stronger unwanted effects, and at worst it becomes a matter of surviving the cure. A study on the various versions of sugar damage of diabetes sums up the best scenario. (Currie, 2010).

Leaving diabetes untreated means high sugar, low insulin and high risk. Treating it with medications brings sugar down and insulin up. This divides the risk between moderately high sugar and insulin, respectively. If one is driven too low, the other one goes up like a sea-saw increasing the risk. However, none of these options stop the disease progression. Only lifestyle will. This study has caused endless confusion in the research community since we cannot give up our blind faith in medications.

Does it Have to Be?

Does it have to be this way? It did not use to be! If we watch TV shows from just fifty years ago, people look like bean stalks. They were normal size. We no longer fit into air airplane seats, and a size small is large.

A woman on TV recently lamented the food industry and its unscrupulous destruction of our health. Another one blamed the government for our destructive food policies. Then a group of bantering TV anchors made cute of their candy-habits.

We are looking for some higher power to save us from ourselves, but that is not in the cards.

It would take large scale political and public health efforts that are not on the radar despite the back-breaking costs of our failure to act.

The kind of progress needed here does not typically come from our fearless leaders. It comes from people who think differently and express it. This oftentimes leads to being ignored, silenced or called worse than daft. Luckily, chances of being burned at the stake are small these days.

But there is More—

We are now clued in to the fact that eating can trigger inflammation. What else can be a trigger?

You have heard it before, but maybe not in this context: Exercise! Or rather, lack thereof—

CHAPTER 4
How We Move

We Are Movers and Shakers

We are natural movers if not shakers, equipped with a resilient musculoskeletal system to support an active lifestyle. Originally, we had no choice in the matter. We had to run faster than dinner, or we would not eat. The ancient Greeks valued physical fitness to the point of inventing the Olympic Games. They treasured their gymnasium, literally meaning a place to exercise naked, while offering a chance to share gossip and socialize.

Our lifestyle throughout history required physical strength, and activities such as competitive stone-throwing became a mandatory part of a decent Viking job interview. We still have residuals of this emphasis on physical prowess in various strength-testing, including competitive wood-chopping, cable-tossing, modern weight-lifting, not to mention the resurrected Olympics. As we became more bookish, these skills fell in value. We have evolved into a culture that works in sedentary settings while placing ourselves geographically and technically so that we can get around without much effort.

Around 1970, two out of ten Americans were in sedentary jobs. By year 2000 almost half Americans were mostly sitting at work. Our culture of watching television reinforces this lifestyle. Not to mention the drive-in restaurants, banks and movies. The combination of our Western diet and this cultural inactivity has ended up causing major health problems. We might indeed say that overweight makes us ill, and sedentary lifestyle adds insult to injury.

Use It or Lose It

Our muscles are powerhouses of protein, made to move, and to move us for that matter. Their shape and health depend on being used, giving meaning to the saying "use it or lose it" because nowhere is this truer. We know this because if we immobilize a limb for days, it will start to atrophy. This is not lost on hospitals. Whatever the illness, the patient is encouraged to stand or walk every day. Early physical therapy is an integral part of restoring the patient to previous functional level, if at all possible. Activity makes us physically stronger and healthier. Yet we are not taking advantage of this wonder remedy. We have a new epidemic: sedentary lifestyle.

The Dangers of Inactivity

The health benefits of exercise were described in medical writings some 250 years ago. Incredulously, an English physician, William Heberden, described a patient who cured himself of angina pectoris by chopping wood. This is not the first choice of activity that a modern physician would prescribe for such a patient, but in this case, the subject apparently lived to tell about it. Anyway, the idea of the connection between activity and health was not pursued and further explored.

Consequently, when overweight started becoming a problem in the latter 1900's, we looked at it largely as a vanity issue. Exercise was promoted for cosmetic reasons in fitness centers and athletic clubs.

As we began to see the wave of chronic illnesses, we realized that inactivity was part of the problem. Once we made the connection between weight and health, the flow of information exploded. The list of dangers of inactivity extends across all our organs and parameters, resoundingly confirmed by studies in major medical journals and health agencies. A sedentary lifestyle is as dangerous for our entire body as smoking. Advancing age and sedentary lifestyle increase inflammation.

Here is a laundry list of health risks of inactivity: elevated blood sugar, diabetes, high lipids, high cholesterol, obesity, heart disease, stroke, sudden death, high blood pressure, elevated inflammation in the body, increased risk of cancer, particularly colon and breast, bone loss, increased risk of osteoarthritis and hip fracture, weakening of the immune system, poor balance, cognitive decline, depression, dementia and Alzheimer's disease.

If this list looks familiar, it is because it is more or less identical to that of high blood sugar and other stressors. Inactivity can cause as much inflammation to the brain as to the body. Some studies show it a stronger predictor of overall mortality than weight.

Exercise Reverses those Dangers

The effects of exercise are so wide-ranging that they cannot be duplicated by any other trigger.

Study upon study shows extensive benefits of exercise on the body's cell systems, be they cardiovascular, bone and muscle, endocrine, immune system or brain.

The result is enhanced strength and function including cognition, stress coping, memory and academic performance. Strong muscles maintain the mechanical tension necessary for an active lifestyle, balance and bone strength. Exercise is antiaging. It is also a mood elevator, effective against depression and attention-deficit by working through natural opioids of the brain. It strengthens our balance, posture, bones and it makes us look better to boot. Like blood sugar, exercise shows a liner relationship with health and life span.

Look Ma, No Pills!

This is such a neglected landmark study of our pill-loving culture that it deserves its own billing. A 2002 study showed that lifestyle changes, including 2.5 hours of exercise per week, was more effective in reversing diabetes than pills. This comes as no surprise since pills just mask the problem.

But How Does Exercise Really Work?

Why is exercise so powerful? Research shows that it has something to do with our very genome. We carry around a paleolithic genome formed by a world of the survivors who ran faster that dinner.

Our genes for metabolic regulation were laid down under those circumstances and encroach on all physiological regulation, accounting for our genetic intolerance of inactivity, as well as dietary and other toxic triggers. Exercise is a trigger that activates the genes for better regulation of insulin and oxygen uptake, metabolism and muscle strength. Adding it all up, it is connected to the inflammatory chain, being antioxidant, anti-inflammatory, antiaging, muscle-strengthening, immune-strengthening and protective against chronic disease.

Inactivity slows down the pathways of the brain and weakens the immune system by direct effect on pro-inflammatory signaling. Muscle atrophy makes us physically weak and slows metabolism. This keeps the ingested sugar from being used, raising our blood sugar. It proves difficult to keep our blood sugar normal without exercise. Diabetes carries a staggering 65 percent increase in risk for Alzheimer's, and even persons with pre-diabetes are at high risk. Unsurprisingly, these risks are lowered by exercise.

This is reflected in our morbidity and mortality statistics. It should give us pause to pick up our jog shoes and take a hike.

Exercise Is a Game Changer

Let us look again at a list of medical benefits of an active lifestyle:

1. Weight. Exercise is a big variable in the energy balance between weight and nutrition. Weight or BMI is not the whole picture. BMI, or body mass index, was invented for epidemiologists and other researchers as a tool to describe large populations but is not necessarily applicable to each individual. "Normal weight" depends on frame and muscle mass. The point here is that a well-trained man with high

muscle mass might register elevated weight or BMI and be perfectly lean and healthy.

2. Cardiovascular disease. The heart is the pump responsible for increasing blood flow as needed, increasing nutrients and oxygen to the body and the brain during higher demand. This builds up the muscle, stamina and cognitive ability while removing toxins and waste from all systems.

3. Diabetes mellitus. This is the prototype of inflammation because insulin resistance is the mother of most chronic disease. Exercise has marked anti-inflammatory effect by lowering sugar, insulin, thereby lowering fat and inflammatory markers. With a good nutritional plan, it will reverse diabetes type 2.

   It needs to be pointed out that diabetes type 1 is the opposite insulin problem. The body cannot produce any, and this comes with another set of problems.

4. Cancer, especially breast and colon. Many cancers start by inflammatory process, and exercise may reverse the inflammation before the development of cancerous transformation.

5. Bone/muscle health. Building up muscle increases metabolism and strengthens physical capacities. Sedentary lifestyle may cause muscle atrophy, stiffness and joint compression. An active lifestyle exposes muscles to mechanical stress, strengthens them and triggers bone formation with increase of bone density. This improves alignment and liberates joints.

6. Improves life quality, strength, prevents falls. Balance, along with muscular exercises, increases coordination, avoiding falls and injuries.

7. Longevity. Exercise has been shown to be an independent predictor of quality of life and longevity, self-esteem and resilience by being in control of our everyday life.

8. Mental health/mood. Exercise lowers blood sugar, clears the brain of inflammation, increases brain cells and increases

mood, protecting against degenerative brain disease including Alzheimer's disease. Body exercise is brain exercise.

As we will see in chapter 5, the CDC lists exercise as a major benefit with respect to academic achievement.

Researchers who work with Alzheimer's came up with a list of risks for this devastating illness, implying that it is a multifactorial disease. Guess what is on that list? The exact risks of sedentary lifestyle.

You might have noticed something else striking. The list of risks for Alzheimer's is literally a copy of the list of risks associated with high insulin, sugar and inflammatory diseases. Furthermore, the list of benefits of exercise is the inverse of that list. This is a reminder of the presence of a unifying common pathway of signals, the basic role of inflammation and our holistic nature. In terms of triggers, harms or benefits, what affects one affects all. The body functions as one big cell.

One Positive Might Not Be Enough

Here is why one beneficial factor alone might not work by itself, regardless of how well we eat. Without the increased rate of metabolism furnished by exercise, it is very hard to get our blood sugar down to zero disease-risk at fasting blood sugar 80 mg/dl, as projected by some studies. When we eat right and also exercise, both lower blood sugar.

What Is Exercise?

When we led active lives, no one had to think about these things, but physical activity has become the subject of scientific scrutiny and description. Throughout history we have inadvertently performed many major clinical studies to give us some pointers.

It turns out that the benefits of exercise are cumulative. If we have an active lifestyle in general, it all adds up. Another interesting thing about exercise is that it seems to be what we make it. The work done by hotel room attendants in a shift qualifies easily as an activity, but studies show that many who do this fairly demanding work do not think they get enough exercise. When they are told that their work, in fact, is exercise, they improve their health compared to a control group by measured standards, such as weight and blood pressure, again demonstrating the power of our brain to help create our experiences.

Lack of exercise along with obesity are now leading causes of disability among young people. A 2001 call to action to all from the surgeon general to become more physically active went nowhere.

People are encouraged to get out of their cars, but our environment is not necessarily designed for foot traffic. The bicycle is gaining in popularity, but there are not enough paths to make cycling safe. Most of all, we have become creatures of comfort. There is our inertia against doing what is good for us because it takes effort. Even walking the stairs or park the car at the far end of the lot is not a common habit. We look with big eyes at the handicap space next to the door. An active lifestyle is no longer the norm, and the change from sedentary to active is not easy or natural.

Muscle Might

We are only as strong as the weakest muscle in the group, meaning we need to exercise all muscles, or we will end up in imbalance.

We have two basic different types of muscle fibers: the slow twitch muscles that do most of the daily work within the limitation of available oxygen (aerobe). In short bursts of energy (resistance, weight-lifting), the muscle recruits the fast twitch muscle fibers and may run out of oxygen after a short time to become less efficient before it stops working (anaerobe).

There are three phases of contraction of the muscle: concentric, or flexion toward the center of the muscle; isometric, or holding the muscle still while loading it; and eccentric, which means slowly lengthening a muscle keeping it under tension.

We now have technical definitions of exercise types based on how the muscle is worked, like this one, published by Harvard Medical School. It divides exercise into four categories:

1. Aerobic exercise. This is an overall cardiac, respiratory and muscular workout. This method uses the large muscles, including the heart muscle, to build health and condition, i.e. heart and breathing rate. A heart rate above 85 percent approaches anaerobic and cannot be sustained because our body cannot deliver enough oxygen at this level. The body takes to burning fuel much less efficiently while accumulating toxic waste such as lactic acid.

2. Strength or resistance training. Using weights to load the muscle makes it work harder, and repeated concentric movements adds work. With proper technique, including full range of movement of joints and muscles, this will strengthen individual muscles and increase muscle mass. Weight-bearing exercise is considered beneficial in the prevention of osteoporosis or low bone mass. The purpose is to put tension on muscles and bones, which promotes bone mineral deposit. However, more weight and fewer repetitions may be deleterious to joints such as knee and shoulder. Isometrics recruits all available motor units of the muscle and is a strength exercise, but do not develop flexibility. It is usually a component of a strength-promoting program.

3. Flexibility. Emphasis on stretching through full range of motion of a joint or muscle rather than load. The purpose is to maintain or increase range of motion and to allow all joints and muscles to move freely. Repetitive motions add strength without wearing on the joints. Keeping the body limber counteracts stiffness and pain. Oftentimes combined with resistance training for strengthening.

    The three previous categories dealt with the muscular system. This last one enters a different territory:

4. Balance. This is the function of a coordinated system made up of receptors in muscles that receive information on where we stand, so to speak; the vestibular apparatus of the inner ear that judges position, kind of like an attitude indicator of an airplane; the eyes integrate the above and adjust for terrain and distance. All these cues from our environment are constantly funneled to the brain and interpreted to hold our core muscles in attention and keep us grounded.

This system is very much a "use it or lose it" system and vulnerable among other things to stress and age. The good news is that much like our muscles, it does respond to being challenged. It is therefore paramount that we exercise this function, and there is a whole set of designated balance exercises to do this. Balance training is any movement that tilts the body out of the line of gravity: asymmetric weight-bearing, reducing of the platform of the body, such as weight shifts, single leg stands, tai chi, yoga and eccentric exercises using our limbs as levers.

Speaking of Eccentrics

For those familiar with our gym culture, we went through the high or low-impact aerobics class, boot camp, spinning, abs, CrossFit, powerlift and various other specialty classes to work on one area or the other. Many of the high-charging routines targeted specific areas and were not necessarily good for us in the long run. We ended up with imbalances and injuries. This has led to a search for alternatives.

Enter eccentrics. This is a form of exercise that deserves more attention. It was introduced by a certain Adolf Fick in 1882, and like many other good ideas, it was subsequently forgotten.

As referenced by Lindstedt, an eccentric muscle action is the slow extension of limb while contracting its muscles, leading to overall lengthening of a muscle as it develops tension. When load exceeds the force that can be developed by the muscle at constant length, as in an eccentric muscle action, the exercise is referred to as involving negative work because the muscle is absorbing energy. This "negative" movement can create more force and lead to stronger muscles than concentric actions while using less metabolic energy.

If we, in addition, stretch the muscle slowly while keeping it relaxed, it will lengthen, if only microscopically lengthening the leaver. In so doing, it will acquire disproportionate amounts of strength when loaded. Relaxing is the new power workout! If this sounds too good to be true, for once it is not. It is the physics of our marvelous muscles.

Eccentrics is making a comeback championed by TV fitness experts like Miranda Esmonde-White, backed by medical science. It is weight-free, using the body and the limbs as levers. Eccentrics also works with the body in a holistic manner, i.e. with full range of motion of chains of muscles from head to toes, stretching, strengthening and lengthening entire chains at a time. Actually, it looks holistically at the body as one big muscle in need of training all fibers equally. This type of regimen has proven effective while avoiding gym injuries. It is excellent all around for muscle strength, flexibility, balance, musculoskeletal rehabilitation and maintenance.

Vanity Can Be A Good Thing

To a certain extent, vanity is a positive and can be a life force. The motivation for looking good can have unintended metabolic benefits. A downtown San Francisco bar gets into the discussion with the following sign: Exercise makes you look better naked, but so does tequila. Just remember that the latter may carry a hefty price tag in the long run.

Exercise—What Kind, How Much, and How Long?

Recommendations in terms of time spent per week is 2.5 hours or 150 minutes, and reaching the total is cumulative.

The working definition of exercise is activity that raises heart rate. Maximal heart rate is calculated by the following equation:

220 minus your age. If you are forty years old, your maximal heart rate would be $220 - 40 = 180$. We divide exercise into mod-

est, high and low intensity. Working heart rate at low would correspond to less than 50 percent of maximal heart rate, modest would be 50–70 percent, and high intensity would go up to 70–85 percent.

Ambling about and its equivalents are low-level activities, which are good for well-being but do not build up cardiovascular status. Walking, jogging, cycling, swimming, dancing and cross-country skiing all fall under moderate activity. Moderate training is effective cardiovascular training when done consistently. A hallmark of this level is being able to talk in full sentences. Intensive training is jumping rope, weight-lifting or playing any sport that causes shortness of breath when talking, and is effectively done in shorter spurts.

Mind-Body Interventions

Driving home the point of our holistic nature, these health-altering modalities straddle activity and thought, emphasizing their confluence. Modern life is oftentimes more about mental than physical pressure, and our thoughts are in a race to juggle everything it has to process.

All the negative triggers we have discussed so far can actually change the way our genes function and tilt us toward illness. Like pure exercise, body-mind practices are triggers that can affect health by lowering inflammation in the body. They are called mind-body interventions and include modalities with or without physical activity, such as yoga, Pilates, tai chi and meditation.

If this sounds like having something to do with our thinking, and energy fields, you are right. Focusing on a simple activity brings us brain rest. We know that thought energy can enter the inflammatory chain and reverse the expression of stress-inducing genes. The energy of inward focus of meditation, perhaps combined with simple movements, might explain the mitigation of the inflammatory response in either form of activity. This adds a whole group of ways to change the neurocircuitry of the brain to our advantage.

Are There Any Downsides to Exercise?

It is hard to come up with any argument against something proven as powerful as the benefits of an active lifestyle, but we will play devil's advocate.

If we think of physical labor as exercise, we know that chronic heavy lifting and overweight may lead to arthritis; repetitious work to overuse syndromes, and fatigue may lead to acute and chronic injuries. This can cause joint compression and damage. Physical laborers and athletes oftentimes have degenerative arthritis and a host of injuries to their extremities such as elbow, wrist, knee-tendon and ligament damage, shin splints, plantar fasciitis and so on. There is evidence that people who do high-intensity aerobic exercise in gyms over many years may suffer injuries or overuse syndromes, but we are also beginning to look at the very training methods being used. We are beginning to wonder about the "no pain, no gain" mantra.

The people who built the pyramids in Egypt had clear evidence of severe wear and tear or degenerative bone problems, just as super athletes may suffer long-term consequences of their top performance over time from musculoskeletal problem to brain damage. We can conclude that lifting two-ton blocks of marble or being knocked in the head repeatedly is not good exercise.

Overweight people benefit from exercise but stress their joints in so doing. One pound of extra weight loads these joints with some four pounds of extra weight. The solution is unweighted water aerobics or the use of especially unweighted cycles or other machines. Exercise is for everyone.

Preventing injuries hinges more on understanding one's musculoskeletal limitations than the dangers of exercise per se.

Studies show that elite athletes, when compared with their sedentary counterparts, lower their lower mortality risk by some 80 percent. This tells us that there is no such thing as too much exercise. The better shape we are in, the longer our lives. What is there not to love about it? I think we lost this argument.

We Have Issues

Other issues might get in the way. There is not much room or incentive for exercise in our lives unless we paddle a bit upstream. My patients used to tell me about the job, the shopping, the family, the PTA, the repairs around the house, the endless to-do list and the late evenings at the office. We are tired, and it is hard to get beyond the must-do's, never mind seeing that we might feel less tired if we exercise! What is a person to do? We need public health and political intervention, but there are ways we can tweak our daily routines.

Lifestyle changes do work. If we walk up a set of stairs or through a long parking lot several times a day, it adds up. If we can find the time, our new lifestyle could be based on a hobby. For instance, if you like dancing and music, surely there is such a workout in a gym near you. Walking and socializing? Friends can be great motivators because we tend to mimic them. Enlist a walking buddy or get a group together, stop at an interesting spot in your neighborhood, or finish with a social at a coffee shop (sans pastry). So be a buddy or seek one out. If you hang around with active people, chances are you will take their cues and become active yourself. Your chances of succeeding are best if you do something you think is fun, so find something fun and do it!

We have now dealt with two of the most important influences on our health: nutrition and exercise. But our environment is full of triggers that go under the radar, and can become health problems unless we recognize and manage them. Our own thoughts are one such group of major triggers.

CHAPTER 5
What We Think

Plasticity Becomes the Brain

According to medical dogma, the brain was a small organ with a formed genetic blueprint that grew into a large one to run our life. It turns out to be the other way around. We are born with immature brains carrying a certain genetic inheritance that gives us predispositions, but this general blueprint starts changing right from the start by responding profoundly to the environment.

Development starts at birth within our families and continues through interactions with our schoolmates, peers and the rest of our surroundings. Positive energy such as visual, motor, tactile, auditory experiences, even exposure to odors, are superior brain builders. Conversely, social rejection and isolation are negative influences capable of decreasing brain size and function. The more secure and supportive our relationships, the more stable our view of ourselves and the world.

There are several stages of development before the brain reaches adult size at about age eighteen. Childhood play is the development of social skills in a complex environment. This is fundamental, because later we see life through a filter of early forgotten events, emotions and learned values, the summary of our experiences.

The most important factor for our brain health and development including intellect is so surprisingly simple it is not really appreciated: positive interaction with the environment, meaning support and nurturing. Lacking this benefit, the brain might take to manifesting chaotic functioning, causing mental or somatic health problems. Even prenatal stress may lead to mental health issues such as ADHD, learning issues and depression. The brain can grow or shrink and change in a matter of minutes depending on how we treat it, and continues to react to the smallest of stimuli throughout our lives, sometimes with unexpected results. This malleability of the brain by the environment is called brain plasticity. It allows us to change and learn all through life.

Being the Brain

The brain is divided according to complexity of task. It collects incoming information and makes the final decisions about how this is integrated and used. Without specific reference to anatomy, the lower part or brainstem deals with vital functioning, including state of consciousness, while middle centers deal with emotions. The upper part of the brain, the cortex, houses the intellect. It decides things from how we learn the tango to writing dissertations.

Remember, we are pattern recognizers. The brain programs itself by building a database to compare new information to old, and delights in forming patterns out of the chaos of stimuli coming at us 24-7. This memory bank evolves with each new bit of information. Learning creates more learning because we use existing knowledge to deduce ever-more complicated ideas. Stepwise we develop language, art and science.

One of the most extraordinary human features is our capacity for abstract, original and creative thinking. The brilliant ideas pushing evolution did not happen overnight; they sprang from that very bank of stored patterns. Standing on the shoulders of our mentors we can take the next step, even turn to the metaphysical world to add new ideas and concepts. Children who grow up in positive environments develop quickly. On the other hand, a child from a neglectful orphanage is unlikely to excel in science music or poetry. In fact, it may even die. A child growing up in the dark would actually be blind if the sensory organ of the eyes were not used, just as a child who did not hear a spoken word would not develop language. This puts an enormous responsibility on us in terms of the experiences we provide for our children. This reality has landed with a thump on our doorstep and has strengthened our interest in brain plasticity and epigenetics.

We Think with Our Gut?

As we mentioned earlier, the gut flora is a key player because it produces the neurotransmitter serotonin, thus establishing "the second brain" and the "brain-gut axis" involved in a number of brain functions, including sleep, behavior and mood. This makes it a factor in the development of mental disorder. It then follows that disturbed integrity of gut flora may produce any illness from colitis and diabetes to depression. Conversely the opposite flow in this system may cause gastrointestinal disorders from "nervous stomach" to colitis. The age-old idea of gut feeling is neither new nor far-fetched.

We Think with the Immune System?

Since half of our immune cells are found in the gut, we have a microbiota-immune-neuroendocrine system, or axis that communicates using molecules that regulate brain and immune function through the gut. It acts as a hub for crosstalk between the brain and the immune system, aided by messenger molecules. These link thoughts to the immune system, which decides what to do with the message.

A strong immune system strengthens our brain capacity, and our gut flora influences both. This confirms the redundancy principle of these connections and should come as no surprise. Damage to any link can cause malfunction through the entire chain, causing mental and somatic inflammatory disorders flowing in any direction. This again shows that the system running our health is supremely holistic.

The Brain Is Emotional

An extraordinary human feature is our complex emotional nature. We typically think of ourselves as rational creatures with the cerebrum or upper brain as the center for critical thinking, and the depths of the mid part being the site of our emotions. Our superior brains have ever intensified these attributes. We sometimes apply our superior brainpower to personal philosophical issues. We are, in short order, capable of extremes like becoming haters and mass murderers. There is nothing rational about harming people who don't think or look like us, but we are capable of the complexity of thought and have just the abundance of molecules to do this.

Molecules of Emotion

In her pioneering work, Dr. Candace Perth showed that signals from the outside can trigger molecules that are recognized by their receptor in a brain cell and assigned a meaning, negative or positive. A plethora of such molecules help create the nuances of sensation. Our thoughts can also generate these molecules. The antennae for these processes are opioid-type receptors.

Dr. Perth showed that all our body cells have these receptors. Our mind is present in all our cells, and thoughts release molecules that influence the genes creating our health. Dopamine is a hormone of movement, and lack of it may cause Parkinson's disease. But it also regulates survival, motivates us to eat, reproduce and experience it as pleasure to boot.

The strong motivation and reward mechanisms that keep our species going also harbor the potential for addiction.

Subtle Effects Count

The brain is like a sponge, absorbing even the most subtle clues in the environment. It has been shown that persons who hold a warm drink in their hand think of others as more friendly. If you want your kids to clean their room, a whiff of cleaning fluid may be more effective than nagging.

Women are thought more attractive dressed in red. Did you ever hear about the song "Lady in Blue"? And just think of how you feel when someone starts sharing their latest litanies of health problems, pain, medications and procedures. Not to mention if they share a juicy story with you. The only thing more contagious than measles is mood.

The Dueling Brains

We might say that we live in an ongoing tug-of-war between the rationality of the neocortex and the reward system of the so-called limbic system, popularly known as reptilian brain.

Dr. Paul MacLeod described this system in 1952. The psychoanalyst Clotaire Rapaille coined this term, studying our desire-and-reward responses. He predicted our so-called reptilian response to consumer products. In the service of the ad industry he used various psychological modalities such as regression therapy to access our memories and uncover subconscious motivations for what we want. The results were convincing.

Among other things, he helped design one of the most successful cars ever, the PT cruiser. We get rewards from spending money on what our reptilian brain thinks we must have. As a result, we buy things we cannot afford and do not need. The PR industry is partly built on these principles, and we are its cultural petri dish.

We are under constant financial and consumer survey by commercial interests that make us consummate shoppers, slaves to our subconscious material desires. This is a step on the road to addictive shopping, gambling, or otherwise. Dr. Rapaille famously said, "The reptilian brain always wins." He had a point.

Addiction

Addiction lives in the lower or reptilian brain. It is a reward system on steroids, so to speak, since it amplifies the addictive message.

We have discussed addiction to edibles. In addition, its ingredients run the gambit from chemicals such as opiates, cocaine, alcohol and nicotine to behavior such as gambling and shopping, that stimulate the reward hormone dopamine, producing a feeling of well-being above normal, called euphoria.

Endorphins are the main transmitter substances inhibiting pain by blocking the sensation of suffering. The sum of it all is a feeling of intense pleasure so great that when the opioid effect wanes, the reward mechanism kicks in seeking another fix to reproduce the feeling.

Natural opioids can be triggered through thought and physical activity, "runner's high," but the easiest way is to take a trigger substance or a form of opioid itself, such as morphine, heroin or synthetic opioids. The brain develops tolerance to the substance and we need higher doses to reach the reward.

When the reward pathways become so hardwired that there is no contest from rational elements, addiction occurs. This is a form of destructive learning, and we fail to learn from our mistakes. It may happen very fast, as we have seen lately. Some of the hallmarks are craving, binging, tolerance and withdrawal. The drive to repeat the pleasure is so strong that it can distort a person's value system and spawn antisocial behavior including crime. This makes addictive substances so destructive.

Treatment of addiction is notoriously difficult. Once those pleasure pathways are laid down, they are difficult to unlearn. This should give us pause to consider the tragedy to individuals and the cost to society of addiction. It also should tell us that it is easier and more cost effective to warn people of addictive substances than luring people into using them. An ounce of prevention is truly better than a pound of cure. In fact, the willful addiction of persons should carry criminal punishment.

The Brain Makes Mistakes

The subconscious is not well understood. It can surface in the strangest places and in unexpected ways. The brain starts laying down experiences in our subconscious before the age of six. They become like hardwired tapes that it uses for judging future situations. Some of our emotional responses are thought to be driven by early childhood experiences where we felt threatened and our responses saved us.

The problem is that both the experiences themselves and the responses might be based on misinterpretations and can be triggered by apparent trivialities. This behavior can be nonproductive, even destructive. It has been said that the conscious brain acts while the subconscious reacts. It is in this subconscious realm we find our most interesting behavior. Child psychologist Alice Miller writes about "lost childhood feelings" that were never expressed and resurface in distorted form often as neuroses or other mental problems.

We are not aware of our subconscious functioning, and we rarely recognize it. The much-cited example is the disproportionate reaction of rage to a tube of toothpaste left without the lid. Such a minor incidence is thought the trigger of a long-forgotten incident that might have nothing to do with toothpaste.

Since the root of such behavior is largely hidden from our view, it is hard to both recognize and change. It has profound implications because it means that the programming of our brain is truly at the mercy of our environment, and the smallest experience can lead to long-lasting alterations in brain growth and development.

It also leaves us open to error because there might be a mismatch between our internal model and reality. We sometimes put these scripts back into the control center and rerun them just to make sure because it is the final authority dictating our behavior. Once the brain misreads or distorts a script, the second reading might be no better than the first. A simple illustration: if we are bitten by a dog, we might think dogs are dangerous and, by mistake, fear all dogs unless we learn differently. The mind has been misinformed to begin with but has recorded it as gospel. It is buried in our subconscious and hidden from us, surfacing only when a trigger situation happens.

The Misprogrammed Mind

Consequently, if we are told we are sickly, we might just live that way because we believe it, and miss out on life because of what could be called software errors in our brains. As we will see under healing, ancient medicine recognized the value of making sure our cerebral software programming is tuned as positively as possible.

We are back to the concept of signal flow. Everything discussed here is framed by our previous discussion of the nature of energy and our place in the universe. It brings credence to the idea of the therapeutic value of mind-energy-based interventions such as mantras, placebos and meditation, and they will be presented here as they are found in mainstream research.

Body-Mind Interventions

Historically we have categorized meditation, hypnosis, homeopathy and acupuncture treatment as quackery. Yoga and other Oriental mindful movement disciplines did not fare much better under the scrutiny of our linear, evidence-based lens. Remember, we know differently because we have documented body-mind interventions. They may work as combinations of the placebo or positive energy reprogramming, empowering the subconscious brain, lowering stress level, strengthening immune responses and ultimately reducing inflammation. It is generally accepted that yoga and breathing exercises can influence our physical as well as our mental health.

Aside from the more obvious stressors, becoming more urbanized and losing touch with nature is now a recognized risk, leaving us more prone to negative health consequences. As we revel in our built environment, we are suffering from stress and lack of brain rest in our daily life.

A new spin on an old body-mind intervention practiced in Japan is "forest bathing," though it involves no water. We call it a walk in the woods. It is the immersion experience of ambling through vegetation enjoying the sounds, smells and scenery. It appears that this activity lowers blood pressure, heart rates and other stress-related ill effects by lowering the stress hormone cortisol. The same calming effect is seen from having a pet. For all of you who have enjoyed the serenity of nature or the beneficial company of our fellow animals, this should come as no surprise. It speaks to the harmony of including everything in the flow. It does not speak so well for our record of destruction of biomass and ridiculing "tree huggers." We are losing nurturing energy from the flow faster than we can register it, and with it the healing interaction with nature itself. It truly is our loss.

The Mind Is Linked-In

In our mathematical description of the brain, we pointed out that it is the physical site of our mind. It only makes sense that it would influence the body by way of energy fields. The phenomenon of quantum entanglement shows that sub-atomic entities under certain circumstances will change the state of the system even remotely, leaving the door open to universal interaction. The mind is the ultimate quantum system. It is an open network of energy fields throughout the body and the environment. This gives it the ability to interpret and respond to signals from everywhere. What we think might have an impact on our neighbors, people across the earth, the environment and the state of the planet. All points are linked in one energy flow, and our self comes from our relationship with it.

The Placebo Effect

We have assumed that when it comes to improving our capabilities, "trying harder" would bear fruit. It speaks to rational behavior and work ethics. Interestingly, the discipline-laden, perhaps even inadequacy-laden message to work harder will make us more tired rather than more capable.

What improves our capabilities seems to be a positive message to boost our confidence that we can. If we fully expect to be able to do something, our mindset can change our brain and, in fact, direct our body chemistry to fulfill on that expectation. This is known as the placebo effect, meaning that we can change our abilities by changing our thoughts. Sound familiar?

A well-known study shows the effect when people are told that pilots have excellent eyesight. They are then put in a pilot's seat of a simulator and actually see better. Hotel maids lose weight and lower blood pressure, but only after being told that their physical work is exercise. We also have a plethora of clear evidence that our thoughts influence our health in medical settings. The response may be emotional, such as feeling less tired or depressed, or it might effect physiological changes, such as lower pulse or blood pressure.

From the same study we learned that people who drank liquid caffeine became stronger. As the caffeine was slowly removed, people retained their strength. Also, when people received injections of growth hormone their hormone level increased, but here is the interesting thing: after a while the level increased even when they were injected with a dose of water. This type of study has been done many times with medications, and repeatedly they show that the brain and body remodel themselves according to what we believe will happen. The placebo principle is known and much used in many contexts. It was validated by men like Henry Ford, who said, "Whether you think you can do something or you don't—you are right." It seems he was right.

This could be seen as showing that the power of positivity as well as that of negativity is self-fulfilling. Both explainable by the science we discussed earlier.

Placebo in Medicine

Across time and cultures we find the healer, "the one who will please," who, for lack of other means, literally works with the way we address the subconscious. At the core is the expectancy and belief that the patients will get better because they believe they will. People have benefited from this sort of help through the ages. Medicine has deemed this "sham' and "dummy" use of remedies with no known effects. Since we have just seen how the placebo connects with our subconscious, this attitude seems a tad, shall we say, outdated.

A paper in JAMA 1955 reported on the treatment of post-operative pain with placebo and consistently showed from 35 to 85 percent pain relief. We mentioned our understanding of the chemical pathways of pain above. Pain can be described as the subjective feeling of distress from physical or mental injury. Astonishingly, the more severe the pain, the more effect of the placebo. The results persisted whether the patient knew or not. In fact, the effects were so great some patients developed side effects of the treatment, so-called nocebo or negative effects. It turns out that placebo works on the endorphin-releasing mechanisms, creating the same dampening effect as opioids on pain as well as euphoria. Numerous studies have confirmed that the placebo effect is consistent across physically and mentally caused pain, as is the nocebo effect.

The opioid crisis has forced a recent interest in placebo, since we are at a loss to treat the epidemic of opioid-addicted patients that we have created. Placebos turn out to be very effective, sometimes combined with less addictive anti-inflammatory drugs. We are still missing serious efforts to take advantage of these observations.

The creation of the opioid disaster literally used opioid as a placebo to create pain to begin with. There is no evidence that we all of a sudden had these masses of undertreated pain patients in this country. There is, however, evidence that "customers" were told that if they were in pain, they needed opioids. This only helped to discredit the use of placebo and derail serious evaluation of its effects.

The most stunning placebo effect shown in modern medicine is probably Dr. Moseley's study on arthroscopy of the knee in arthritic patients. It showed that whether the patient had surgery was not key to their post-operative quality of life. The fact that they believed they had undergone the procedure was the deciding factor. It rocked the world of medicine, and we might say it shows that if you look, you find, and vice versa.

Mind-Bending Mantras

Mantras are the repeated concentration on, or chanting of, the same word or phrase to literally implore our brain to install a pattern of thinking. It has been part of Eastern spiritual life for thousands of years and has found favor in the West for its calming and positive effects through words association and the hypnotic cadence of the repeated chant.

The world of advertising uses it so successfully there is no need for proof of whether it works. It does so by reinforcing a message of reward for following the recommended advice, be it buying or doing something. We see these incessant repeated messages when we turn on our TV set. It is classical conditioning or learning by repetition, in short, reprogramming our brain.

In extreme cases, using mantras could be called brainwashing. Our response is feeling good about this message and thinking we need the intervention in question. As with placebo, we don't need an intermediary; we can tailor auto-suggestions to ourselves, internalize the message to become a script that we follow without realizing it. The directive can be used to motivate ourselves to regain control. It is clear that we can if we approach the brain where it listens. It is our loss that we are not tuned in to this resource.

Research has shown mantras to create new connections in the brain. We can interrupt negative thoughts and create new positive ones in their place. The working theory of their effect is the energy vibrations created by the repeated chant. After all we have learned about our nature, this is confirmation that our thoughts influence energy and that energy influences our thoughts, creating our reality where we chose to focus.

If we give up the idea that the body is simply a machine with fixable parts, health becomes a matter of our entire energy field controlling the equilibrium of the body. We also know that mind and matter mutually influence each other without being linked by physical conduits. As we have discussed, the energy flow is multidirectional, and a particulate matter, such as an edible or exposure to other toxins, can cause mental-health changes. We see the melding of the body and mind and the blurring between somatic and mental illness.

Whether or not we acknowledge this holistic concept, it is at work around us. Once we know that any type of interpersonal stress, anger and social rejection are strong risk factors for depression and illness from asthma to stroke, we have to fall back on the nonlinear explanation that our health status is an overall balance of our collective energy fields.

If this is so, we should find the immune system a clearing house for all manner of negative energy, expressed as inflammation. We should also find that mental, as well as somatic diagnoses, are inflammatory in nature and respond to anti-inflammatory medications. Studies are suggesting that this general mechanism holds true.

We Need to Be Linked In

While we lamented the epidemics of obesity, smoking, inactivity and social stressors, we discovered another health risk we have already alluded to: loneliness. Social isolation has been identified as a major risk for mental as well as physical health in young as well as old. Research is finding that growing old alone doubles the risk of illness and early death, equaling or surpassing that of overweight. As Americans grow older, there is a loneliness epidemic looming. Some forty-five million older Americans are suffering from loneliness.

This speaks volumes to our failure to understand the holistic model of the mind presented above. We need to be connected and feel part of our surroundings. This is a system where all points are connected and can influence each other over distance.

Loneliness is expressed as feeling isolated without meaningful relationships to our fellow human beings. It is a most negative force, and engenders thoughts that are inflammatory in nature.

As a society, we are becoming less social and more virtual in our communication. This discourages meaningful closeness and nurturing. Considering that these are more important to brain development than intellectual stimulation, this is a worrisome development for our mental capacities and to our health in general.

The dangers of being left outside the flow of the universe are repeatedly confirmed, sometimes in the most brutal manner. Disconnectedness from the greater society is a recipe for pathology in younger men. They connect with groups who feed into their negativity. The profile of school shooters and serial killers is often that of disconnected and isolated individuals. Living in a world where violence is the norm is detrimental to us all. All changes, positive or negative, affect our own functioning and that of the whole system.

Brain Foods?

Like the rest of the body, the brain needs high-quality food to function optimally. The Centers for Disease Control has a very informative website called *Health and Academic Achievement*, which provides evidence-based information regarding the connection between academic performance and access to healthy food and physical activity.

The assessment was done on grades, behavior such as attendance and drop-out rate, as well as cognitive skills, concentration and mood. All were linked to the amount and quality of food, down to specific nutrients and vitamins. Physical activity proved equally important. This is a reminder that a treat is not necessarily a treat, and a ringing endorsement of school breakfast/lunches and PE. It has led to the latest slogan in popular medicine: brain food. It implies that the brain is a separate organ, which is exactly what it is not.

Aside from being 2/3 water, it consists of more fatty acids than protein; and like all cell walls, those of the brain contain cholesterol. Protein and essential fatty acids of the omega-3 type are crucial building blocks, causing fish oil to be considered brain food. A variety of supplements are thought to be brain-growth promoting. For instance, a diet high in choline has been shown to reverse stress in rats around the time of birth. The point is that a nutrient-dense diet has decisively been proven to prevent inflammation and is a major determinant in brain health, while major studies link sugar with depression and other mental-health issues.

With the sugar/obesity epidemic, we see an avalanche of brain disease at both ends of life when we are the most vulnerable. One in five children now carries a mental-health diagnosis, and Alzheimer's disease is a scourge. Both are linked to diet and body weight. It turns out that what is good for the body is good for the brain, and a balanced, nutrient-rich diet is the best health-insurance policy.

The Mind in Health and Illness

We have now seen that the brain depends on our actions, such as what we eat and how we behave and think. It typically does not create a specific illness "to order", but like any other organ, if it is inundated by negative energy, malfunction will cascade through the system and create inflammation and illness. We associate certain illnesses with stressful thoughts, well known examples are ulcers and cardiovascular disease.

We saw earlier that psychological stress can increase our risk for stroke. The *San Francisco Chronicle*, August 31, 2016, featured "illness tied to high rents in Oakland," naming asthma, high blood pressure and anxiety. A massive display of the power of the brain over bodily matters is heart disease from the stress-related heart attack to the so-called Tako-tsubo, or broken-heart syndrome. This latter is a brief episode mimicking a heart attack and causing acute, though reversible, heart failure. It is typically experienced by people without known heart disease, but with a history of profound psychological stress.

Chances are that, even thinking ourselves invincible, we might not be guaranteed good health if we abuse it in some respect. We see throughout this book that there is more to good health than good thoughts. It makes no sense than three-hundred-pound persons with diabetes could think their way into good health. Rather, we need to create positive energy flow by moderating all aspects of our lifestyle. In short, chances are that we have to be good stewards of all our gifts for the universe to meet us halfway.

CHAPTER 6
Where We Live

This is the fourth slice of the health risk pie. Traditionally, health risk related to our geographic location has been relegated to environmental medicine. With the increasing recognition of illnesses as the interface between us and our environment, our geographic situation has become central to the discussion of illness in general.

We might start by remembering this:

We Are Not Alone

We already introduced our smallest cohabitants, the microbes. We recognize their beneficial role in the gut and the potential damage of their infectious variety. In reality, they have helped shape our history and their imprint looms large.

They are ubiquitous, meaning they are everywhere. Each of us is host to a stunning hundred trillion of them, some thirty trillion more than we have body cells. Beneficial microbes are overwhelmingly more numerous than pathogenic ones, but the few that cause human disease can be all the more malignant. Since their lethal potential and mode of transmission were not understood for centuries, there was no treatment. Many microorganisms may use insects or other animals as intermediate host or vectors. Infectious conditions can kill, scar or disfigure for life.

Microbes have shaped our world and determined the rise and fall of kingdoms. Historically, societies were ravaged by epidemics including plague, smallpox and tuberculosis. Infectious diseases repeatedly played a decisive role in world-altering events such as the decline of the Roman empire under emperor Justinian. They decimated armies and weighed in on battles, notably the Peloponnesian wars. The great plague of Europe killed around twenty-five million people. Some 90 percent of native Americans were wiped out by viruses including smallpox, measles and influenza.

Microbes Are Fighting Back

The discovery of antibiotics ended the ravages of many bacterial epidemics, a major milestone in medicine. While these remedies are not always available in underdeveloped countries, they are so overused in the West that it is becoming a problem. Microbes learn to overcome antibiotics. They keep up with our ingenuity to become "superbugs" that are antibiotic resistant and crop up in the most sterile environments, even hospitals. It is therefore critical to their efficacy that their use be restricted. Antibiotics have been used routinely and indiscriminately for years, treating everything from undiagnosed conditions to fattening up livestock. Predictably, we are now seeing microbes that are multiresistant to our drugs, leaving the door open to new infectious disease epidemics.

While we have eradicated the most common microbial diseases by developing effective vaccines, these prove more elusive for many of the major pathogens, such as those causing the deadly trio of malaria, dengue and yellow fever. Viruses elude most anti-microbials and are proving difficult to treat.

Fire and flooding may change the habitat of pathogens and cause unexpected diseases. Extensive travel has increased our risk of devastating epidemics. Haiti became a dreaded example of disaster aid gone wrong when relief workers brought cholera and death to thousands. Secondary disasters in the form of debris and organic material fomenting epidemics may follow. This is often the case in war zones.

Being There Changes Everything

As we saw in the discussion of quantum theory, we change an environment merely by being there. It is obvious that our presence has radically changed the earth. As we innovate and solve problems, we create new ones that we don't see coming and are not prepared for.

We are relative newcomers here. For millions of years, nature was in its own flow between forces of expansion and destruction. At one point, the top predators were the dinosaurs who ruled by brute force and lack of natural enemies. Though their population was presumably kept in check by a 90 percent mortality rate of their young, this ecosystem was but a link in the chain of evolution of our planet and vanished in time. It is unclear who ruled after their demise, we think they were smaller surviving animals that kept developing till we started to see bipeds with enlarging brains. Combined with a growth rate out of proportion with the rest of the ecosystem, these qualities eventually gave us the capacity to truly change the planet.

Our Built Environment

For thousands of years, humans operated in survival mode. Their activities were too small to make much of an impact. Like dots in a vast landscape, the scattered populations slowly grew in proportion to the bounty offered by nature and moved to follow the trail of the next meal. With the appearance of permanent shelters and farming some ten thousand years ago, the idea of crops and food storage started. More people could be fed. When the Catalhoyuk people built their neolithic settlements of mud brick houses in Anatolia and started domesticating animals, they certainly did not understand that they were starting the cultural recipe for a slow brewing crisis thousands of years later. Increased population density led to organized societies of farmland and villages. The same thing was happening in other fertile areas of China and India. The problem was not the amount of activity, but the principle involved. The competition between nature and human development was in full swing. There was no serious impact for some nine millennia. It finally caught up with us and has quickly developed from being the elephant in the room to the urgent existentialist issue it is today.

The Agricultural Revolution

The eighteenth century became the era of exploration of natural sciences. Farming could now be further intensified aided by technology.

While most third-world countries farm at subsistence levels, factory farming is now the norm in the West, presenting a complex nonlinear set of direct and indirect drivers of climate change.

Our forests and greenery are part of the lungs of our planet. Denuding the land and taking the trees out of the ecosystem are drivers of greenhouse gases, as is intensive production of animal protein. Even small-unit farming is a driver of environmental deterioration. It represents a constant loss of land. The use of environmental toxins such as pesticides and chemical fertilizers further the damage, including the loss of pollinating insects and birds. Toxic chemicals pollute soil and waterways, all integral to clean water. This depletes the soil with loss of nutrients and downgrades food quality.

Irrigation technologies altering the flow of water stress the downstream surroundings and cause subsidence of the land. The result is lower crop yield, inability to sustain populations, malnutrition, hunger and the need for more land. The result is all-encompassing damage to the holistic environment, affecting every living system on the planet.

The Industrial Revolution

The agricultural revolution was the perfect precursor to the industrial one. Populations grew and were freed up to seek other work as a transition in employment was spurred on by innovations such as the steam engine. This led to the building of railways and factories. Manufacturing had largely been done in the home by artisans. With the literal explosion of machines, railroads and factories mining transport, mass production became cheap and the need for labor great. The most powerful energy source for this revolution was coal. No thought was given to possible negative effects of industry. The only brake on the process was availability of resources.

The urbanization that followed saw centers of over-crowding and pollution. Factories were located to cities populated by workers who lived in squalid conditions of poverty, child labor was rampant. High density of built structures traps heat, raising temperature. Concrete surfaces prevent runoff and increase risks of flooding. Loss of nature's green lungs made them hubs for climate change and global warming. Inadequate waste disposal caused toxic environments and slums. Industrial pollution became so high that the air would be darkened by smoke and other pollutants.

Carbon Boom, Planet Bust

The carbon era started when the industrial revolution turned into an unprecedented technological one that is still booming on the basis of three major ingredients that made it possible: the fossil fuels of oil, coal and natural gas. As mentioned, coal was the first significant polluter, but the high energy use made possible by the burning of oil and gas products added the production of what we call greenhouse gases. They are the main culprits in our planetary woes.

Land loss combined with our fossil fuel industry cause the depletion of resources while creating large amounts of toxic waste that turns air, soil and water into ever more contaminated environments. Mountains are demolished mining for raw materials. Refineries spew out a mixture of nitric and sulfuric oxide and other toxic gases, along with particulate matter, ozone and dirt, creating smoke or smog. This toxic gas layer traps heat and warms the air, which again causes changes in the behavior of wind, weather and climate.

High levels of toxins, such as carbon dioxide (CO_2) and sulfur dioxide are gases that condense and precipitate as acid rain destroying plant life. They also dissolve in water, acidifying the ocean and freshwater alike. All these developments brought several unanticipated consequences that are with us on an ongoing basis. They all stem from the single common source of fossil fuel, feeding the rising temperature on earth known as global warming.

We Are Losing the Ocean

Though we treat it as our universal garbage can, the ocean is one of our greatest resources in terms of climate and valuable protein food. Algae produce oxygen. One species that thrives in polluted waters is a toxic alga called "red tide." It depletes oxygen and concentrates poison, killing fish and birds. Along with increasing carbon dioxide and temperatures, this is killing the coral reefs, the natural home and food resource for untold species of marine life.

We are blithely dumping millions of tons of garbage a year into the ocean, including toxic chemicals, fertilizers and plastics, poisoning aquatic life by starvation, suffocation or pollution. Destruction of fresh water, fish habitats, extinction of species and the appearance of new parasites follow. The ocean is overfished and impoverished. While the sea is our main source of essential marine fats, we have rendered this reservoir so polluted that seafood may be dangerous to our health. We give no thought to the fact that what we dumped will at one point appear on our plate. Rivers, lakes and other small reservoirs of fresh water are losing their runoff from melting ice packs, harmed by acid rain and being diverted for irrigation. We are already seeing shortages of potable water. Water encompasses 70 percent of the surface of our planet, and incidentally 70 percent of our bodies. Wholesale poisoning it only shows our appalling lack of understanding of its importance for the holistic cycle of life.

Plastic or polyethylene is a compound with longer half-life than radioactive substances. It is broken down into small particles, appearing throughout the eco chain including our bodies, and clogs up the oceans and beaches, suffocating marine and bird life. We have no idea of how to deal with it, yet we keep it coming.

The start of a most nefarious practice happened in Northern California in 1946 when some fifty thousand drums of radioactive waste were dumped into the waters around the Farallons, a bird and fish sanctuary outside San Francisco. The practice was perpetrated by the Atomic Energy Commission and supposedly ended in 1983. For good measure, a ship loaded with radioactive material was sunk there in 1951. This led to the worldwide practice of dumping nuclear waste in the world oceans. Nuclear waste dumping in the ocean is still going on, whether it be a continued practice or accidental. The consequences of this on public health in the Bay Area and elsewhere are unknown and unaccounted for.

Global Warming

Global warming is caused by the trapping of heat in the atmosphere.

We breathe oxygen or O_2. It plays a critical role in our energy metabolism while producing the waste product carbon dioxide, or CO_2. One man's garbage is the other's gold: reversing this process, plants and the sea use CO_2 to produce oxygen. They are rightly called the lungs of the planet. The two processes keep each other in check, the object being to keep our temperature stable, our air clean and our planet livable.

But what happens if one speeds up while the other one slows down? This is exactly what is happening.

We spew out CO_2 while the shrinking forests and poisoned oceans cannot reverse it to oxygen. The rising temperature with all its consequences is called climate change. Our CO_2 producing lifestyle has made us major emitters of this heat-trapping gas

The principle is that warm sunlight hits the earth. This heat is partially absorbed, partially bounced back into the atmosphere. At this time, our atmosphere contains the highest levels of CO_2 on record, and acts like a blanket trapping the heat. The production of carbon dioxide is at full throttle while the removal system is dwindling. The loss of this CO-removal mechanism by deforestation, denuding of land and polluting the ocean has skewed the balance to cause global warming, also called the greenhouse effect on our planet. The temperature on earth keeps rising in increments. It does not seem like much, but here is the problem:

Just like us, our fellow travelers in the ecosystems are extremely sensitive to temperature. The smallest change influences the entire chain and may cause damage from loss of soil, fauna, flora and marine life to displacement or extinction of species.

The holistic chains that keep natural processes in balance are broken, and the result is the breakdown of our entire biosystem.

Global warming is melting our ice reservoirs on our mountains and in the polar regions, raising the ocean levels, already causing flooding of parts of our landmass including several pacific islands and cities such as New York, Tokyo, London. We are seeing loss of the earth's air-conditioning, temperature increases and steadily worsening wildfires.

The Health Consequences

As the cities became hubs of human density, conflict, stress and crime appeared. So did rampant disease. The list of toxic elements produced by our modern society is lengthy and includes a litany of compounds toxic to the environment and to the development and health of our body and brain.

Industrial areas where these compounds are often processed become contaminated. They are often located to economically depressed areas. This may lead to high incidence of illnesses called clusters. The neighbors who suffer harm from them might not have the resources to protest their presence, and so they are not studied and removed.

Some infamous examples have reached the world press, such as the herbicide poisoning of the village of Bhopal in India, the history of exposure of soldiers in Vietnam to Agent Orange with its resulting cluster of cancers, and the malicious poisoning of the drinking water of Flint, Michigan by city officials. The recognition of the 9/11 New York firemen's syndrome brings home the toxic effects of fires burning structures and building materials.

Noise, even light pollution, can cause health problems including lung disease and stress disorders. Air pollution includes dust, fumes and small particulate matter that cause allergies or chronic inflammation and cancer.

We cannot necessarily connect the accumulated health effects to specific diagnoses, but we can relate risk to environment. Once we use statistics, the numbers do just that.

Microbes may cause compound damage in overwhelming disasters with high mortality, destruction and inadequate cleanup. The WHO estimates that 50 percent of the world's population is at risk for infectious diseases, many of which are opportunists that become pathogens when they come together with other social ills, such as crowding, poverty and poor sanitation. Because the West has a vigilant public health system, we depend on it to stop epidemics from happening. Quite coincidentally, it is being put to the test at the time of this printing with the scourge of the new corona virus pandemic.

Location, Location, Location

Statistics from CDC, 2019 on leading causes of illness and death in the US showed heart, lung and other chronic disease including cancer.

On the other hand, the list of deaths in third-world countries per WHO, 2018 included infectious and diarrheal disease.

The results speak clearly of accumulated stress in widely diverging environments rather than genes.

This drives home the point of illness being overwhelmingly environmental. Some five million die a year from poisoning by contaminated water. Some 50 percent of the world's population are at risk for diarrheal disease caused by contaminated water and infections. Some 30 percent are malnourished.

The idea of geography-related health risk is so clear that it has been studied at the local level, and a surprisingly nuanced picture has emerged. Our health can be predicted on the basis of our postal code, in fact, on the basis of our street address. Poverty is a negative health predictor with its often-attendant low quality housing in high-traffic areas, lack of basic education, poor life skills, opportunity and toxins in the ambient environment.

These findings have led to the concept of geomedicine. It emphasizes the influence on our health of every environment we have lived in. This information should be considered part of our health history, thus inform diagnosis, further care and recommendations.

While interesting in terms of diagnosis, geomedicine might be more effective if used preventively rather than descriptively. The implications are that, applied early and proactively, it could change the course of the patient's health. This would take medicine out of the office, including recommending the removal of patients from harmful environments. Health risk maps are not readily available, but the real limitation of this approach would obviously be socio-economical.

Long-term Consequences

Global warming and climate change will become health risk equalizers if the predictions of the Center for Disease Control and Prevention have any merit. As the deterioration of the planet goes on, our health will be tested in many ways, including increasing loads of cardiovascular disease and respiratory diseases provoked by heat and toxins. New infections carried by air and water will surface. Crowding and loss of space and sustenance will cause mental health issues, injuries, malnutrition conflict and fatalities.

The American Medical Association and the American Heart Association just joined forces with those declaring climate change a health emergency. This is a nonpartisan effort, backed by several other large medical associations, acknowledging that millions of Americans have already been affected and it is time to act. It takes the situation out of the realm of the suffering polar bears to our doorstep where it belongs. Needless to say, if we understood what is good for us, we would have come to the aid of the polar bears long ago. We should not be indifferent and fooled by geographic remoteness, because it is not possible for us to separate ourselves from what is happening. We are all subject to the universal effects of holistic laws.

Win the Battle, Win the War?

When it comes to the impact on our ecosystem as a whole, CDC has published a chart that integrates the effects of rising temperatures throughout its spheres. It reiterates the interconnectedness of our life with all other forms of life and forces, and what happens as the system is thrown off balance.

Unsurprisingly, these conditions include increased CO_2 and extreme heat leading to increased air pollution, changes in insect habitat, pollen, allergens, desertification of land, loss of crops, migration, melting of ice caps, rising sea level water contamination, malnutrition, flooding, fires, weather extremes, general environmental and nutritional degradation.

We would do well to add continuing pandemics to our list. The renowned zoologist and disease ecologist Dr. Peter Daszak, president of the Eco Health Alliance, was instrumental in pinpointing the origins of SARS. He has been warning us for years of the appearance of new and more serious epidemics. He seems to have a point. As temperatures change and we encroach on their territory, microbes change their attack strategy to evade our interventions, and are becoming ever more difficult to fight.

Our entire ecosystem is an enormous biome of humans, plants and animals living in balance with unknown numbers and species of environmental microbes, of which some form our gut microbiome. Everything in the biome competes and changes, driving evolution through its exposure to each other and the environment. Any organism will respond to imbalance by adapting. We now recognize that viruses are a major driver of human evolution. Just as we see the unbalanced gut biome cause illness, environmental microbes will express new genetic information, causing the emergence of new forms including harmful ones. Epidemics have functioned as sporadic checks on our population numbers, but we have learned to limit them while we are becoming ever more numerous, meaning more pressure. Our accelerated population growth is a fundamental stressor.

The Unmentionable

We know that periods of global warming alternate with periods of cooling, called hot house and ice house periods. We also know we are on the hot house track. However, this normally takes millions, not a few hundred years. So what is different this time? Us. We are the only species whose numbers are not subject to systemic ecological regulation while equipped with an innate biological drive to procreate. We are also the species that has caused the current list of calamities while being of no known benefit to the planet. Quite to the contrary, any improvement to our lot destroys the home of others and alters the web that keeps the planet healthy. This unbridled expansion is now showing its effects.

By some scientists we have exceeded the planet's carrying capacity by some five-fold. Our exceptionalism has kept this view taboo. In response, we have created this myth that we can tame nature. We are going to build ourselves out of the deluge of the rising seas with walls around our most valuable real estate such as New York and other big cities. We want economic security and creature comforts for those of us who can afford to live inside the wall. What good will this do if we lose our planet's lungs and air-conditioning and destroy its soil and productivity? Call me a naysayer, but call me in ten years.

Furthermore, we have put the problem on its head, thinking we can "create resources" as the planet runs out. This is tantamount to the philosophy of palliation in medicine. While treating the symptoms, we are not removing the splinter, and the result is inevitable: fix one, another one leaks.

For all our valiant efforts it cannot work because we are dealing with the ultimate holistic system and its built-in inevitability. Which also dictates that the planet itself will take care of the problem. It has already started by bringing a steady stream of disasters to all continents.

Is it All a Hoax?

So why do so many people believe all this is a hoax? This reminds me that, for years, we could not get patients to take their blood pressure medication, not to mention change their lifestyle, because they could not feel or see high blood pressure. It is called denial. This works till the accumulative damage catches up with us, and we have a stroke, heart attack or other acute event. We are dealing similarly with other inconveniences in life because they cramp our style, that is, our reward system, a bit. We want it all now, we want instant gratification. We denied the damage caused by nicotine for a long time. We know that obesity will eventually cause us problems from arthritis to diabetes, yet we don't feel sick and we neglect to change our health while there is time. With respect to global warming, we are now seeing acute proof that the patient is ill if we are willing to look.

Quantum Entanglement

If we don't believe in eco-science, we are, in effect, ignoring our quantum nature. Recall that the universe is a flow where all points are connected in an energy field. Each point can influence another anywhere in the universe, and the energies can reinforce or weaken each other at any distance.

As we mentioned earlier, our mind commands energy. Thoughts and actions can change the flow. One action, positive or negative, can cause reactions on a nonlinear basis in any direction and along any pathway and change the system. The impact is open-ended, a small input can lead to large, unpredictable changes. This might manifest now or in the future. We are all connected over space and time.

Historically, people intuitively understood this. They had rituals for removing negative energy. Once we recognize this, we can see how important it is for the health of the system that its energy stay positive. Health, then, is not needing spare parts, but an energy flow through the entire system. The health of the energy field determines the message, thus the health of the system. That is the law.

What's Love Got to Do with It?

We have worked through four chapters to get to the point: Our health and why we get sick. We started out challenging the common belief that illness is something that arbitrarily visits upon us, and that we deal with at the doctor's office. We ended up in eco-science. How we take care of the environment determines the quality of our air, water, food and, as we have seen, even our serenity of thought. If you remember nothing else of this book, remember this: Our health is informed by our communication with each other and with the universe. The most important communication is positive energy. That would be love. We are talking the ethical idea of universal nurturing rather than dating. Well, then again, it is a fact that a bear hug has bona fide healing effect. In case you think this comes from a San Francisco philosopher, I hasten to include the reference source: The Harvard school of medicine.

This makes love serious business. By respecting and loving our fellow beings and our home we bring healing to all. This is true quantum power.

We Are All in This Together

Or are we? The COVID 19 crisis has revealed that some of us are more in it than others. The virus has unmasked the disparities of our social system. We have created a corrosive and divisive world where the least resourceful bear the burden, and potential talent and resources are being squandered through small-mindedness. Our income and opportunity inequalities are glaring from the images of hungry neighbors and grim health statistics. This is counter to Lamarck's observation that we humans represent the pinnacle of evolution through cooperation and inclusiveness. It defies the idea of a positive, healing universe and weakens us as a whole. We are now seeing some consequence of this. It finds us wringing our hands at the idea of redistributing our resources to benefit all, and is only hastening our descent into, oh well, as not to offend you, I will let you fill in the blank.

The Health Risk Pie

This completes the health risk pie.

We are routinely bombarded by health gurus who tout "the one thing we have to do to be healthy." The reality is that everything we do triggers changes in how our genes work. The resulting action changes the environment, which in its turn changes our gene function, forming the mutual interaction between genes and environment that shapes our lives. The circle is complete. Our choices will cascade through, adding to the final outcome of the ecosystem and reverberate back to us through generations.

The message is that we can have our pie, but careful how we treat or eat it! It will at all times define our collective health and that of our home here on earth.

CHAPTER 7
Healing

Our Hellenistic Heritage: Asclepios

My Greek vacation was in many ways a real eye-opener. We met a people visibly under siege by austerity and social problems, but their inner grace and spirit were equally visible. They showed us honesty and dignity we thought no longer alive in the world. Besides, I walked through my history book, meeting up with Electra and Nestor alike. While this is not a travel log, Delphi was truly the navel of the world.

But my most unforgettable experience as a doctor was walking into the sanctuary of Asclepios in Epidaurus. This was the most famous healing center of the ancient world, built around the cult of the healing god Asclepios. I literally walked into the world's first hospital and the dawning of modern medicine from ceremonial healing to physical modalities. Despite limited scientific understanding, their thinking around medicine was extremely advanced and pragmatic, and the museum on the premises attests to that. The hospital was state of the art and included a village of temples, baths, sports arena, totaling accommodations for 1,400 patients and families. All built to the highest classical standard of beauty that has served as a beacon of architecture ever since. Located on a hillside in the beautiful valley of Epidaurus, it was a haven of harmony and tranquility.

They Started by Using Placebo

When the patients were admitted, the Aesculapian priest/physician started the therapeutic process by calling on their inner resources through ceremonial appeals to their own healing energy. They would drink from the sacred stream that ran across the sanatorium grounds, then take their place in the sleeping hall. In their dreams, Asclepios himself would visit them and offer advice on what they should do to get well. This is the highest form for calling on your inner spiritual healing energies through placebo.

Since you have read the preceding chapters of this book, you now understand that forces including the healing mechanisms of the brain and the immune system can be unleashed by the energy at work. The appeal to these resources may come in the form of rituals, potions, verbal assurances and expectancy. Whatever form, they represent positive energy flow that enables and may unleash profound effects on biological systems, including measurable changes in neurological pathways and energy-state of the body. We also know that, like modern medical spas, they took therapeutic advantage of the nearby mineral rich springs from which the stream originated. Whether or not the patient would go on to need further treatment, they now had their own inner energies mobilized. If the patient's inner resources were not curative, the treatment progressed with diagnostic and even invasive procedures.

They Did Trauma Care

We know from their advanced instrumentation that they did not expect to remedy tumors and repair injuries with ceremony; they proceeded to do surgery. Their sophistication is again on display. Standard surgical instruments were invented here, and surprisingly, few improvements have been done to their basic form. Though rooted in cults to gods we cannot subscribe to, modern medicine might take note of the way treatment was dispensed in a stepwise fashion, involving the patients practically and spiritually in their own cure.

A Complete Holistic Approach

The idea of the hospital as a village and the importance of a living community functioning and worshipping with the patient is also revolutionary. This suggests an understanding of our connectedness and the value of nurturing during healing, not just forgotten, but outright contraindicated by western medicine until relatively recently. For instance, some sort of misguided modern authoritarianism dictated that children were not to see their families while in the hospital for fear that they might get upset. Many a case of post-traumatic stress came out of that philosophy.

The theatre featured plays, and the stadium and gymnasium encouraged exercise and competitions such as chariot racing, clearly involving society at large. Within their limitations they even understood the importance of good hygiene, dedicating this important domain to the goddess Hygiea, daughter of Asclepios, and giving rise to the saying that cleanliness is next to godliness. This was nascent public health and limited only by their lack of understanding of microbiology.

Hippocrates

Aesculapian medicine was so successful that other hospitals were built, among them the Asclepion on the island of Kos along the Turkish coast. This is where the physician Hippocrates is said to have trained. He built on the Aesculapian model of holism, emphasizing the connectedness of patient to the environment. He introduced record-keeping and set standards as well as ethical rules for treatment and professional conduct. His system of medical practice became the paradigm for medical care in the western world. Some of his writings have survived and serve as the basis for the so-called Hippocratic Oath that is considered a standard in the profession today.

Testimonials from the Thankful

The records left by the Asclepians including Hippocrates tell us that they used the spectrum of modern modalities including art therapy. They emphasized the participation of the patient in good eating, exercise, supportive care and positive thinking.

If this is beginning to sound like the message of this book, it is no accident. Despite the lack of understanding of modern science, ancient Greek medical practice was more complete than ours and in a modern setting would probably have been far more successful because they understood the importance of treating the person as a whole. We are now beginning to look backward, recognizing a spiritual component to illness and the importance of self-help, community and family in healing.

We know they were successful despite their limited resources. The walls of the hospital in Epidaurus are replete with votive tablets, often depicting the body part that was healed, along with testimonials to the effectiveness of the treatment.

Whatever Happened to Primum Non Nocere?

Modern medicine is a marvel of high-tech rescues and procedures, and we are all glad it is so. We are scientists, approaching health in ever-more high-tech fashion. However, medicine has strayed from its Hippocratic roots of seeing the patient as a whole.

Here is a contradiction: Medicine is "evidence-based," whatever that means, since the evidence is that we don't cure, but offer relief from symptoms rather than addressing the underlying process. But as we have seen, more lifestyle treatment raises the risk of complications. With the rise of modern medicine, we forgot Hippocrates in anything but name. This runs counter to the foundations of medicine to which we swear allegiance: first do no harm.

We, the Scientist Healers

Most ancient cultures including all European ones have a history of ritual healers, but their approach was not that sophisticated. In fact, our own was pretty gruesome until fairly recently and included arsenic and other poisons. As spirituality waned and science overtook medicine, the idea of calling on our inner healing forces lost credibility to the scientific approach.

We have a culture of scientists who cannot see past their microscopes and can only discuss these matters from that vantage point. Our singular faith in science-based medicine has led away from the spiritual aspect of illness and to the hegemony of the pharmaceutical industry. We turn the diagnostic process on its head when it suits us. We even invent studies and diagnoses to accommodate drugs.

Holistic medicine is at best thought of as idealistic but unrealistic in our busy, sophisticated world. What is the evidence, since we cannot collect accurate data points? Has holistic medicine ever been tried on a large scale, and did it have any merits? We have just learned that yes and yes; it is, in fact, the foundation of Western medicine-

Our Health Is Cosmic

We have seen throughout this book that diseases are rooted in process, not parts. If we are stuck in the linear lane fixing symptoms rather than addressing the underlying processes, we cannot fully understand them. We need the quantum dimension to see the whole.

Both our power-generating energy metabolism and the signals transduction are fraught links where the process can be thrown off balance by matter energies.

This means that in the holistic world, our health is in a constantly changing equilibrium with the environment. We cannot separate ourselves from it because it is our source, our trigger. We end up in a balance between its many facets: our genetics, stress load, support system, coping resources but most of all, our behavior. Good health can then be described as the convergence of all the energies discussed here into positive flow and the absence of negative energy or stress.

Once we see this entanglement, it becomes evident that our health is not a simple end point of a stream of pills. Going to the doctor and expect to be "fixed" in a visit might not work.

While we treat the body largely on a physical level, we already use energy fields to treat certain skeleto-muscular and mental health diseases. It becomes only reasonable that we understand illnesses as holistic networks of processes, and feasible that the two could be integrated and complementary.

Healing Is Reversal

Since we have repeatedly shown that our health is largely at the mercy of our environment, it is our challenge to approach it in a healing mode, not just a palliative one.

Understanding illness as a function of negative triggers of the immune system, we have choices. We can stop damage by removing the triggers, thereby shutting it off. We can further use the power of our minds to create a different reality by calling on our healing forces to create good health.

This is where all medical camps fall short.

It does not make any sense that one could counteract the damage of sugar or air pollutant poisoning by energy manipulation. If we fail to remove the toxin, the problem by all logic would continue. While it seems a good thing to meditate while eating sugar, it would be rational to remove the sugar and reverse negative processing by meditating. And perhaps throw in some exercise. Not to mention kindness to others and the planet. Recall, negative energy is inflammatory, connectedness is basic to healing, and energy is cumulative.

Following this logic, we become the picture of strength and health once all our energies are in positive alignment. This is not space-cadet gibberish; it is the consequence of our being part of the universal energy.

The Big Question

A big question is how far our healing power goes. This is unproven territory because it cannot really be quantified in studies.

The power of the brain is touted as all-healing as long as we fervently believe we are well, but this reasoning falls short since persons who do not even understand they are sick do die.

Without understanding the limits of this power, it would be reasonable to think that we can remove triggers to restore ourselves as long as we are in reversible inflammatory stage of an illness, where there is enough viable tissue left to support life.

I yield to miracles.

At this point it must be said that this book is written in context of our present understanding of medical science. However, we are on the threshold of a new brave world that in its utmost consequence could change medicine as we know it.

Created in whose Image?

Meet CRISPR, acronym for "clusters of regularly interspaced short palindromic repeats". This describes pieces of genetic material that allow us to actually edit our genes. We already use this type of technique in the genetic modification of food.

Orwellian as it sounds, we can now delete or change genes, snippets, or single components that we deem undesirable. We can use the same technique to alter the genes of future generations.

By trading out old genetic material, we could then exchange old characteristics for new ones, though this exchange is proving more difficult than a simple removal of unwanted parts.

We hail this as a way to stop or reverse illnesses.

In its ultimate consequence, we can image a supercomputer with every feasible gene edited to its best function and using this template to create our children to order.

We haven't heard much about it, possibly because its implications are a tad overwhelming. Questions arise immediately:

Might genes interact in ways we don't understand? What might be the effects of the genome if we start tinkering with it?

Who writes the template for what is attractive or desirable, and who decides on behalf of the unborn child? Since medical science historically is used as a political tool, who wants to live in a society where this kind of power is potentially available to a despot?

The deployment of these techniques is far away, but the feasibility is there. We would do well to remember that every time we take a leap forward without understanding the consequences, nature shows us surprises we had not thought of, and they are typically on the same scale as our projects.

In the end, we might see a risk-benefit equation that limits our dream of the famous free lunch and direct our efforts back toward shared responsibility for what happens in life. We have a high leap and a long way to go.

Making the Quantum Leap

We have seen all through this book that the development of illness is a complex melding of our body, brain, genes, immune system as energy systems that respond to the onslaught of environmental trigger energies that all flow together to create our lives. There is healing as well as destructive power in this flow. We are one with and inseparable from the universe. What happens to it happens to us.

Our next quantum leap will not be in the discovery of a gene or a machine. It will be the understanding that our lives are the result of the collective message we take down from the environment and, in fact, what we send back into it. The circle is complete. We will always be defined by the part of the flow we call on.

What are you calling on?

EPILOGUE

The last piece of the health pie came like a thief in the night during the writing of this book. All of a sudden there it was, the ominous state of our planet. Every day there is more bad news. Natural forces are unleashed to make people ill, homeless and destroy property to the tune of millions across the continents. I realized that this is our most massive and imminent health threat on a global scale.

I cannot help but feel like the opera composer who ended up weeping over the fate of his heroes and had to write alternate endings because he could not bear to let them all die at the end.

So What Might Be Our Purpose Here, If Any?

If it is to live a constructive life and take care of our common home, we are not the first, just the current candidates to face the test.

Looking into space the way we have been privileged to do lately, it should occur to us how insignificant we are in cosmic terms. We are given a speck of land so small it might not show up on anyone else's radar if they exist. It is also so uniquely beautiful. We can do better than to destroy it.

Can the Universe Feel Pain?

It depends on how we look at it. Our forebears thought so. They did not know modern mathematics or quantum theory, but they understood nature in ways that we don't. They felt our interwovenness, and the idea that pain felt at one point reverberates in the system.

Primitive as we think them, many of them realized that all living cells are intelligent and emotional and that even inanimate objects have existence and purpose. We repeatedly testified to feelings and thoughts of the intelligent cell. All energy of our pain, grief, depression, anxiety and sorrow for the suffering of the world, of the sick, injured, killed and disappeared flows from our brains into the universal river of energy and joins the fabric of the universe as a wave with that of all fellow beings. You might have heard people say that nature is crying. Or rejoicing. Our brains are the transducers of emoting between us and the environment and the two-way mirror between us and the universe. What we call on, happy or sad, will reflect from the universe and back into it since we are its mirror.

Is This Our Luck?

We have seen here that nature offers many pathways of probability that something might happen, inferring that there is no planned reality. It is up to us to shape the energy flow that keeps our holistic system positive, because our health, in fact, our very existence here depends on it. Understanding the detailed theory of this is not necessary to grasp the message of this book. Neither is it really necessary to understand that we could have been rocks floating in the Kuiper Belt.

However, as luck would have it, we are here, given the option to thrive in good health, eat our vegetables and watch the sunset.

Therefore, one final message has to be understood: We create our luck as we go. This carries an awesome responsibility for understanding our luck as outlined here, or it might run out.

BIBLIOGRAPHY

Chapter 1

Darwin, Charles. *The Origin of Species by Means of Natural Selection.* Reprint by Penguin Books, 1985.

Balter, M. "Was Lamarck Just a Little Bit Right." *Science* (2000) 288:38.

Newton, Isaac. *The Principia: Mathematical Principles of Natural Philosophy.* University of California Press, 1999.

Spencer, H. *Principles of Biology* (1864). Reprint Creative Media Partners LLC, 2019.

Twain, M. *The Gilded Age: A Tale of Today.* Penguin Classics Reprint, 2001.

Watson and Crick. 1953. "A Structure for Deoxyribonucleic Acid." *Nature* 171: 737–738.

Bygren, L., Tinghog, P., Carstensen, J., Edvinsson, Kaati, S., Pembrey, Sjostrom, G. M. 2014. "Change in Paternal Grandmothers' Early Food Supply Influenced Cardiovascular Mortality of the Female Grandchildren." *BMC Genetics.* 15:12.

National Institute of Diabetes and Digestive and Kidney Diseases (NIDDK), part of the National Institutes of Health. Report Aug 2017.

CDC Health, United States. 2017. Table 53 pdf icon [PDF—9.8 MB]

Cloud, J. "Why your DNA isn't your destiny." *TIME Magazine* (2010) 18: 49–53.

Stephen, M., Rappaport, Rodney, John Scott, Editor. 2016. *Genetic Factors Are Not the Major Causes of Chronic Diseases.* PLoS One. 11(4): e0154387.

Egger, G., *et al.* 2004. "Epigenetics in Human Disease and Prospects for Epigenetic Therapy." *Nature* 429, 457–463.

Morandini, A. C. and Yilmaz. 2016. "Role of Epigenetics in Modulation of Immune Response at the Junction of Host–Pathogen Interaction and Danger Molecule Signaling." *Pathog Dis.*74(7): ftw082.

Kaelin, W. G., McKnight, S. L. 2013. "Influence of Metabolism on Epigenetics and Disease." *Med Oncol* 153(1): 56–69.

Hemminki, K., Lorenzo, Bermejo, J., Forsti, A. 2006. "The Balance Between Heritable and Environmental Aetiology of Human Disease." *Nat Rev Genet.* 7(12): 958–65.

Bird, A. 2002. "DNA Methylation Patterns and Epigenetic Memory." *Genes Dev.* 16 (1): 6–21.

Jacobson, K. *Considering Interactions between genes, Environments, Biology and Social Context. Psychological Science Agenda.* April 2009 (science/about/psa/index.aspx).

Schwanhäusser, B., Busse, D., Li, N., Dittmar, G., Schuchhardt, J., Wolf, J., Chen, W., Selbach, M. 2011. "Global Quantification of Mammalian Gene Expression Control." *Nature 473* (7347): 337–4242.

McLeod, S. A. (2019, May 28). *Introduction to the normal distribution (bell curve).* Simply psychology: https://www.simplypsychology.org/normal-distribution.html

Herrnstein, Richard J., Murray, Charles. *Bell Curve: Intelligence and Class Structure in American Life.* Simon and Schuster, 2010.

Lialiaris, T., Mantadakis, E., Kareli, D., Mpountoukas, P., Tsalkidis, A., Chatzimichail, A. 2010. "Frequency of Genetic Diseases and Health Coverage of Children Requiring Admission in a General Pediatric Clinic of Northern Greece." *Ital J Pediatr.* 36:9. PMID: 20205810.

DeAngelo, M. J., Kish, V. M., Kolmes, S. A. 1990. "Altruism, Selfishness, and Heterocytosis in Cellular Slime Molds." *Ethology Ecology and Evolution* 4: 439–443.

Brian J. Ford. 2012. *The Secret Power of the Single Cell.* Originally published in the New Scientist, 24 April 2010.

Eshel, Ben Jacob, Becker, Israela. 2004. "Bacterial Linguistic Communication and Social Intelligence." *Opinion TRENDS in Microbiology* 12:8.

Boisseau, Romain P., Vogel, David and Dussutour, Audrey. 2016. "Habituation in Non-Neural Organisms: Evidence from Slime Moulds." *Proceedings of the Royal Society of Biological 283 Sciences* (1829): 20160446.

Anfinsen, C. B. 1972. "The Formation and Stabilization of Protein Structure." *The Biochemical Journal* 128 (4): 737–49.

Berg, Jeremy M., Tymoczko, John L., Stryer, Lubert, Clarke, Neil D. 2002. "Protein Structure and Function." *Biochemistry*. San Francisco: W. H. Freeman.

Cunningham, J., Estrella, V., Lloyd, M., Gillies, R., Frieden, B. R., Gayenby, R. 2012. "Intracellular Electric Field and pH Optimize Protein Localization and Movement." *PLoS ONE* 7(5): e36894.

Aoi W and Marunaka Y 2014 "Importance of pH Homeostasis in Metabolic Health and Diseases: Crucial Role of Membrane Proton Transport." Biomed Research International Review Article ID 598986 https://doi.org/10.1155/2014/598986

Squecco R Luciani P et al. 2016 "Hyponatraemia alters the biophysical properties of neuronal cells independently of osmolarity: a study on Ni^{2+}-sensitive current involvement" Experimental Physiology. 101(8) 1086-1110

Wilkins, Marc. 2009. "Proteomics Data Mining." Expert review of proteomics. England. 6 (6): 599–603.

Enright, A. J., Iliopoulos, I., Kyrpides, N. C., Ouzounis, C. A. 1999. "Protein Interaction Maps for Complete Genomes Based on Fusion Events." *Nature* 402 (6757): 86–90.

Blackstock, W. P., Weir, M. P., Weir. 1999. "Proteomics: Quantitative and Physical Mapping of Cellular Proteins." *Trends Biotechnol* 17 (3): 121–7.

Veech, R. L., Kashiwaya, Y., King, M. T. 1995. "The Resting Membrane Potential of Cells Are Measures of Electrical Work, Not of Ionic Currents." *Integr Physiol Behav Sci.* 30 (4): 283–307. Review.

Makela, Riejo. "Living Cells Are Electromagnetic Units." *Earthpulse Flashpoint* Series 1 Number 1.

Foletti, A., Grimaldi, S., Lisi, A., Ledda, M., Liboff, A. R. 2013. "Bioelectromagnetic Medicine: The Role of Resonance Signaling." *Electromagn Biol MedDec* 32(4): 484–99.

Hendricksen, Wayne A. *Transduction of Biochemical Signals Across Cell Membranes*. Essay. Quarterly Review of Biophysics 38, 4, pp. 321–330. Cambridge University Press, 2005.

Jeremy M. Berg, John L. Tymoczko, and Lubert Stryer. Chapter 15: Signal-Transduction Pathways. An introduction to Informational Metabolism. *Biochemistry*, Fifth edition. New York: W H Freeman, 2002.

Chen, W. 2004. "Evidence of Electroconformational Changes in Membrane Proteins: Field-Induced Reductions in Intra Membrane Nonlinear Charge Movement Currents." *Bioelectrochemistry* 63 (1–2): 333–5.

Ross CL. Energy Medicine: Current Status and Future Perspectives. *Glob Adv Health Med.* 2019;8:2164956119831221. Published 2019 Feb 27. doi:10.1177/2164956119831221

Lyn Freeman: Measurement of the Human Biofield and Other Energetic Instruments. Chapter 20 "Energetics and Spirituality" by Dr. Beverly Rubik

Jacobson, Jerry I: A quantum theory of disease, including cancer and Simko, M., Mattesson, M. O. 2004. "Extremely low frequency electromagnetic fields as effectors of cellular responses in vitro: possible immune effects." *J Cell Biochem* 93: 83–92

Kuzyk, P. R., Schemitsch, E. 2009. "The Science of Electrical Stimulation Therapy for Fracture Healing. *Indian J Orthop.* 43(2): 127–131.

Huang, H., Savas, D., Hao, Z., Ferkey, D. M., Pralle, A. 2010. "Remote Control of Ion Channels and Neurons Through Magnetic-Field Heating of Nanoparticles." *Nature Nanotechnology* 5: 602–606.

"Researchers Use Magnetic Fields, Rather Than Drugs, To Control Cellular Signaling." Article, *Science Daily*, Jan 2008.

Cohen, David. "Biomagnatism: Magnetic Fields Produced by the Human Body." Lecture. MIT, Nov 7, 2008.

Rosenberg, Barnett. "Electrical Conductivity of Proteins." *Letter to Nature* (1962) 193; 364–365.

Ganong's Review of Medical Physiology, Twenty-sixth Edition by Dr. Kim E. Barrett (2019)

David P Corey. "Channel Protein Converts Vibrations to Electrical Signal." Summary. *Harvard Medical School* (Oct 13, 2004).

Tsong, T. Y. 1989. "Deciphering the Language of Cells." *Trends Biochem Sci Cell Biology* 14(3): 89–92.

Kringstein, A. M., Rossi, F. M. V., et al. 1998. "Graded Transcriptional Response to Different Concentrations of a Single Transactivator." *EUSA* 95(23): 13670–13675.

Goodman, R., Blank, M. 2002. "Insights into Electromagnetic Interaction Mechanisms." *J Cell Physiol* 192 (1): 16–22.

Siegel, D. 2016. *Mind: A Journey to the heart of Being Human.* WW Norton and Company.

Smith Churchland, P. *Neurophilosophy: Toward a Unified Science of the Mind-Brain.* MIT Press, 1989.

Mayer, E. A. 2011. "Gut Feelings: The Emerging Biology of Gut-Brain Communication." *Nat Rev Neurosc.* 12 (8):10.

Clarke, M. B., Sperandio, V. 2005. "Events at the Host-Microbial Interface of the Gastrointestinal Tract III. Cell-to-Cell Signaling Among Microbial Flora, Host, and Pathogens: There Is a Whole Lot of Talking Going On." *Am J Physiol Gastrointest Liver Physiol.* 288(6): G1105–9. Review.

de Waal, F. *Are We Smart Enough to Know How Smart Animals Are?* New York: W. W. Norton & Company, 2017.

Shi, N., Li, N., Duan, X., Niu, H. 2017. "Interaction Between the Gut Microbiome and Mucosal Immune System." *Mil Med Res.* 4:14.

Clarke, G., Stilling, R. M., Kennedy, P. J., Stanton, C., Cryan, J. F., Dinan, T. G. 2014. Minireview. "Gut Microbiota: the Neglected Endocrine Organ." *Mol Endocrinol.* Aug 28(8): 1221–38.

Pagel, Heinz R. *The Cosmic Code: Quantum Physics as the Language of Nature.* Dover Publications, 2011.

Lipton, B. *The Biology of Belief: Unleashing the Power of Consciousness, Matter & Miacles.* Hay House Inc.,2005.

Henry, R. C. 2005. "The Mental Universe." *Nature* 436 (7047): 29.

Cox, B. and Forshaw, J. *The Quantum Universe.* Da Capo Press, 2012.

Abraham R. Liboff, PhD. 2004. "Toward an Electromagnetic Paradigm for Biology and Medicine." *The Journal of Alternative and Complementary Medicine* Volume 10, Number 1,

Guenter Albrecht-Buehler, Ph.D. Cell Intelligence. http://www.basic.northwestern.edu/g-buehler/FRAME.HTM.

Ingber, D. E. 2006. "Cellular Mechanotransduction: Putting All the Pieces Together Again." FASEB J. (7):811–27. Review.

Goto, S., Okuno, Y., Hattori, M., Nishioka, T., Kanehisa, M. 2002. "LIGAND: Database of Chemical Compounds and Reactions in Biological Pathways." *Nucleic Acids Research* Volume 30, Issue 1, 402–404.

Jim Conroy, Ph D: The Tree Whisperer www.PlantKingdomCommunications.com.

Chapter 2

Bidle, T, McKinley M Dr., O'Loughlin V. Anatomy and Physiology: An Integrative Approach—2nd edition

McGraw-Hill Publishing Company 2nd Edition 2016.

Roitt, I. *Essential Immunology.* Wiley: Seventeenth Edition, 2017.

Cannon, W A Laboratory Course in Physiology, Harvard University Press 6th ed. 1927.

Selye, H. 1955. "Stress and Disease." *Science.* 122 (3171): 625–631. doi:10.1126/science.122.3171.625.

Mattson MP. Superior pattern processing is the essence of the evolved human brain. *Front Neurosci.* 2014;8:265. Published 2014 Aug 22. doi:10.3389/fnins.2014.002

Siegel, Daniel J. Mind. A Journey to the Heart of Being Human. Norton Professional Books 2016

The Philosophy of Alfred North Whitehead. Southern Illinois University-Carbondale Second Edition, 1951.

"Incidence and Prevalence of Chronic Disease." (MPKB)—MPKB. org https://mpkb.org/home/pathogenesis/epidemiology.

Kyriakis, J. M., Avruch, J. "Sounding the Alarm: Protein Kinase Cascades Activated by Stress and Inflammation." *J Biol Chem* (1996) 271(4): 24313–6. Review.

Slavich GM, Irwin MR. From stress to inflammation and major depressive disorder: a social signal transduction theory of depression. *Psychol Bull.* 2014;140(3):774-815. doi:10.1037/a0035302

deFerranti, S., Mozaffarian, D. "The Perfect Storm: Obesity, Adipocyte Dysfunction and Metabolic Consequences." *Clin Chem.* (2008) 54 (6): 945–55.

Reaven, G. 2005. "The Metabolic Syndrome: Requiescat in Pace." *Clin Chem* 51:931–38.

Schneiderman, N., Ironson, G., Siegel, S. D. 2005. "Stress and Health: Psychological, Behavioral, and Biological Determinants." *Annu Rev Clin Psychol.* 1: 607–28. Review.

Stanford University Medical Center. "How Stress Can Boost Immune System." *ScienceDaily* (21 June 2012). <www.sciencedaily.com/releases/2012/06/120621223525.htm>.

Calderon, R., Schneider, R. H., Alexander, C. N., Myers, H. F., Nidich, S. I., Haney, C. 1999. "Stress, Stress Reduction and Hypercholesterolemia in African Americans: A Review." *Ethnicity & Disease* 9 (3): 451–462.

MJ Kenney and CK Ganta. 2014. "Autonomic Nervous System and Immune System Interactions." *Compr Physiol.* 4(3): 1177–1200.

Muller, W. E., Blumbach, B., Muller, I. M. 1999. "Evolution of the Innate and Adaptive Immune Systems: Relationships Between Potential Immune Molecules in the Lowest Metazoan Phylum (Porifera) and Those in Vertebrates." *Transplantation* 68: 1215–27.

Cordain, L., Eades, M. R., Eades, M. D. "Hyperinsulinemic Diseases of Civilization: More Than Just Syndrome X." *Comp Biochem. Physiol* (2003) 136(1): 95–112.

Cinti, S., Mitchell, G., et al. "Adipocyte Death Defines Macrophage Localization and Function in Adipose Tissue of Obese Mice and Humans." J Lipid Research (2005) 46 (11): 2347–55.

Philip, Hunter. 2012. "The Inflammation Theory of Disease. The Growing Realization That Chronic Inflammation Is Crucial in Many Diseases Opens New Avenues for Treatment." EMBO Rep. 13(11): 968–970.

Bugni, J. M., Green, S. L., Lee, Chung-Wei, Pang, B., Borenshtein, D., Rickman, B. H., Rogers, A. B., Moroski-Erkul, C. A., Mcfaline, J. L., Schauer, D. B., Dedon, P. C., Fox, J. G., Samson, L. D. 2008. "DNA Damage Induced by Chronic Inflammation Contributes to Colon Carcinogenesis in Mice." *J Clin Invest.* 118(7): 2516–2525.

https://www.cchr.org › cchr-reports › inventing-disorders › introduction.

Air Pollution Is the 'New Tobacco,' Affecting 90 Percent of All Children. https://www.newsweek.com › ... › Health › Environment › World Health Organization (Oct 19, 2018).

Geerlings, S. E., Hoepelman. A. I. 1999. *Immune Dysfunction in Patients with Diabetes Mellitus (DM).* FEMS Immunol Med Microbiol. Dec. 26(3–4): 259–65. Review.

Myers, Lindsay, MBA, MPH. 2014. *The Self-Help Industry Helps Itself to Billions of Dollars.* Essay, May 23.

Andriote, J-M. "Legal Drug Pushing: How Disease Mongers Keep Us All Doped Up." Essay. *The Atlantic* (April 3 2012).

Wolinsky, H. "Disease Mongering and Drug Marketing." *EMBO reports* (2005) 6(7): 612–614.

Timothy O'Shea, MS. "Pharm D:10 Scariest Prescription Drug Side Effects." *Pharmacy Times* (Feb 01, 2016).

Ghosh A, Ray A, Basu A. Oppositional defiant disorder: current insight. *Psychol Res Behav Manag.* 2017;10:353-367. Published 2017 Nov 29. doi:10.2147/PRBM.S120582

Frick, P. J., Lahey, B. B., Loeber, R., Stouthamer-Loeber, M., Christ, M. A. G., & Hanson, K. 1992. "Familial Risk Factors to Oppositional Defiant Disorder and Conduct Disorder: Parental Psychopathology and Maternal Parenting." *Journal of Consulting and Clinical Psychology* 60(1), 49–55.

Miller, A. *The Drama of the Gifted Child.* Harper Collins Reprint, 1997.

Chapter 3

Elvebakk, R. "The Food Tree." *Amazon* (2008).

Meisenberg, G., Simmons, W. H. *Principles of Medical Biology.* Mosby Books, Inc., 2006.

Robbins. *Basic Pathology Tenth Edition.* Elsevier, 2017.

Centers for Medicare and Medicaid Services 2016–2025 Projections of National Health Expenditures. Data Released Feb 15, 2017.

"Centers for Disease Control and Prevention." *National Diabetes Statistics Report* [Internet], 2017. Available from https://www.cdc.gov/diabetes/data/statistics/statistics-report.html. Accessed 30 November 2017.

Very low-calorie diets. "National Task Force on the Prevention and Treatment of Obesity, National Institutes of Health." JAMA (1993 Aug 25) 270(8): 967–74. Review.

Foster-Powell, K., Holt, S., Brad-Miller, J. 2002. "International table of glycemic index and glycemic load values." *AM J Clin Nutr* 76: 5–56.

Ludwig, D. S. 2000. "Dietary Glycemic Index and Obesity." *J Nutr* 130: 280S–83S.

Thomas, D. E., Elliott, E. J., et al. 2007. "Low glycaemic index or low glycaemic load diets for overweight and obesity." *Cochrane Database Syst Review* CD005105.

Tirosh, A., Shai, I., Tekes-Manova, D., Israeli, E., Pereg, D., Shochat, T., Kochba, I., Rudich, A., Israeli Diabetes Research Group. "Normal fasting plasma glucose levels and type 2 diabetes in young men." *N. Engl. J. Med.* (2005 Oct 6); 353(14): 1454–62. Erratum in: N. Engl. J. Med. (2006 Jun 1); 354(22):2401.

Subar, A. F., Krebs-Smith, S. M., et al. 1998. "Dietary Sources of Nutrients Among US Children 1989–91" *Pediatrics* 102(4): 913–23.

https://www.endocrineweb.com/.../type-2-diabetes/insulin-resistance-causes-symptoms.

Festa, A., D'Agostino, R., et al. 2000. "Chronic Subclinical Inflammation as Part of the Insulin Resistance Syndrome." *Circulation* 102: 42–47.

Nichols, G. A., Hillier, T. A., Brown J Center for Health Research, Kaiser Permanente Northwest, Portland, Oregon. 2008. "Normal Fasting Plasma Glucose and Risk of Type 2 Diabetes Diagnosis." *A J Med* 121: 6;519–524.

Sears, B. and Ricordi, C. 2011. "Anti-Inflammatory Nutrition as a Pharmacological Approach to Treat Obesity." *J Obes.* (2011): 431985.

Aas, A-M, Seljeflot, I., et al. 2006. "Blood glucose lowering by means of lifestyle intervention has different effects on adipokines as compared with insulin treatment in subjects with type 2 diabetes." *Diabetologica* 49(5)872–80.

"America's Health and the Robert Wood Johnson Foundation The State of Obesity 2018: Better Policies for a Healthier America." Report.

Festa, A., D'Agostino, R., et al. 2002. "C-reactive protein is more strongly related to post-prandial glucose load than to fating glucose in non-diabetic subjects; the Insulin Resistance Atherosclerosis Study." *Diabetic Medicine* 19:939.

Cavalot, F., Petrelli, A., et al. 2006. "Postprandial glucose loads a stronger predictor of cardiovascular events than fasting blood glucose in type 2 diabetes mellitus, particularly in women: lessons from the San Luigi Gonzaga Diabetes Study." *J. Clin. Endocrin Metabol.* 91: 813–19.

Hillier, T., Pedula, M. 2001. "Characteristics of an adult population with newly diagnosed diabetes." *Diabetes Care* 24:1522–1527.

Biddinger, S. B., Haas, J. T., Yu, B. B., Bezy, O., Jing, E., Zhang, W., Unterman, T. G., Carey, M. C., Kahn, C. R. "Hepatic insulin resistance directly promotes formation of cholesterol gallstones." *Nat Med.* (2008 Jul); 14(7): 778–82.

Avena, N. M., Rada, P., et al. 2009. "Sugar and Fat Binging Have Notable Differences in Addictive Behaviour." *J Nutr* 139(3): 623–28.

Phelan, S., Hill, J. O., Lang, W., Dibello, J. R., Wing, R. R. 2003. "Recovery from relapse among successful weight maintainers." *Am J Clin Nutr.* (2003 Dec); 78(6): 1079–84.

https://health.gov/dietaryguidelines/2015/…/nutrition-and-health-are-closely-related.

Khaw, K. T., Wareham, R., et al. "Glycated hemoglobin, diabetes and mortality in men in Norfolk cohort of European prospective investigation of cancer and nutrition." *Br Med J* (2001); 322: 15–18.

103. Selvin, E., Coresh, J., et al. "Glycemic control and coronary heart disease risk in persons with and without diabetes: The Atherosclerosis Risk in Communities Study." *Arch Int Med* (2005); 65: 1910–16.

DiNicolantonio, J. J., O'Keefe, J. 2017. "Markedly increased intake of refined carbohydrates and sugar is associated with the rise of coronary heart disease and diabetes among the Alaskan Inuit." *Open Heart.* 4(2): e000673.

Giugliano, Dario, Ceriello, Antonio and Esposito, Katherine. 2006. "The Effects of Diet on Inflammation." *Journal of the American College of Cardiology* 48(4).

Sears, B., Ricordi, C. 2011. "Anti-inflammatory nutrition as a pharmacological approach to treat obesity." *J Obes.* (2011) pii: 431985.

Takahashi, K., Chang, W-C., et al. 2011. "Dietary Sugars Inhibit Biologic Functions of the Pattern Recognition Molecule, Mannose-Binding Lectin." Program of Developmental Immunology Department of Pediatrics, Massachusetts General Hospital Open Journal of Immunology 1:2–49.

Flower, R. 2004. "Lifestyle Drugs: Pharmacology and the Social Agenda." Trends in Pharmacological Sciences 25 (4): 182–5.

https://www.psychiatry.org/patients-families/ptsd/what-is-ptsd.

Laiteerapong N, Ham SA, Gao Y, Moffet, HH. Liu, JY Huang ES, Karter AJ. 2019. The Legacy Effect in Type 2 Diabetes: Impact of Early Glycemic Control on Future Complications (The Diabetes & Aging Study) Diabetes Care 42 (3) 416-426

Després, JP Ph.D. Lamarche, B M.Sc, Hyperinsulinemia and the Risk of Coronary Heart Disease N Engl J Med 1996; 334:952-958

Currie CJ, Peters JR, Tynan A, et al. 2010Survival as a function of HbA(1c) in people with type 2 diabetes: a retrospective cohort study. *Lancet.*;375(9713):481-489

Chapter 4

Owen, N., Sparling, P. B., Healy, G. N., Dunstan, D. W., Matthews, C. E. 2010. "Sedentary behavior: emerging evidence for a new health risk." *Mayo Clin Proc.* 85(12): 1138–41.

"Early mobilization improves outcomes, shortens length of stay in surgical ICUs." https://www.massgeneral.org/News/pressrelease.aspx?id=1994.

"U.S. National Library of Medicine. Health Risks of an Inactive Lifestyle Also called: Sedentary Lifestyle, Sitting Disease."

"What Healthcare Professionals Should Know about Exercise." CME Resource (April 2005); 128(7)3–21.

Pierre-Louis, B., Aronow, W. S., et al. "Incidence of Myocardial Infarction or Stroke or Death at 47-Month Follow-Up in Patients with Diabetes and a Predicted Exercise Capacity 85% vs>85% During an Exercise Treadmill Sestamibi Stress Test." Clinical Study. *Preventive Cardiology* (Winter 2010).

Radiological Society of North America. "Walking slows progression of Alzheimer's, study suggests." *ScienceDaily* (2 January 2011).

Curfman, G. D. 1993. "The health benefits of exercise." A critical reappraisal. *N. Engl. J. Med.* (Feb 25); 328(8): 574–6. No abstract available.

Belotto, M. F., Magdalon, J., Rodrigues, H. G., et al. 2010. "Moderate exercise improves leucocyte function and decreases inflammation in diabetes." *Clin Exp Immunol.* 162(2): 237–243.

Magalhães, P. M., Appell, H. J., Duarte, J. A. 2008. "Involvement of advanced glycation end products in the pathogenesis of diabetic complications: the protective role of regular physical activity." *European Review of Aging and Physical Activity* 5(1) 17–29.

Heberden, W. 1772. "Some account of a disorder of the breast. Medical Transactions." *The Royal College of Physicians of London* 2: 59–67.

Nguyen, L. H., Liu, P. H., Zheng, X., Keum, N., Zong, X., Li, X., Wu, K., Fuchs, C. S., Ogino, S., Ng, K., Willett, W. C., Chan, A. T., Giovannucci, E L., Cao, Y. 2018. "Sedentary Behaviors, TV Viewing Time, and Risk of Young-Onset Colorectal Cancer." JNCI *Cancer Spectr.* 2(4): pky073.

Bonaldo, P., Sandri, M. 2013. "Cellular and molecular mechanisms of muscle atrophy." *Dis Model Mech.* 6(1):25–39. Review.

Warburton, D. E., Nicol, C. W., Bredin, S. S. 2006. "Health benefits of physical activity: the evidence." *CMAJ.* 174(6): 801–809.

Mandsager, K., Harb, S., Cremer, P., Phelan, D., Nissen, S. E., Jaber, W. "Association of Cardiorespiratory Fitness with Long-term Mortality Among Adults Undergoing Exercise Treadmill Testing." *JAMA Netw Open.* Published online October 19, 2018 1(6): e183605.

Vallance, J. K., Gardiner, P. A., Lynch, B. M., D'Silva, A., Boyle, T., Taylor, L. M., Johnson, S. T., Buman, M. P., Owen, N. 2018. "Evaluating the Evidence on Sitting, Smoking, and Health: Is Sitting Really the New Smoking?" *Am J Public Health* (Nov); 108(11): 1478–1482.

Jakicic, J. M., Otto, A. D. 2005. "Physical activity considerations for the treatment and prevention of obesity." *Am J Clin Nutr.* (Jul); 82(1 Suppl): 226S–229S. Review.

Lopez, O. L., Jagust, W. J., DeKosky, S. T., Becker, J. T., Fitzpatrick, A., Dulberg, C., Breitner, J., Lyketsos, C., Jones, B., Kawas, C., Carlson, M., Kuller, L. H. 2003. "Prevalence and classification of mild cognitive impairment in the Cardiovascular Health Study Cognition Study: Part 1." *Arch Neuorol* 60(10): 1385–9.

Kalyani, R. R., Corriere, M., Ferrucci, L. 2014. "Age-related and disease-related muscle loss: the effect of diabetes, obesity, and other diseases." *Lancet Diabetes Endocrinol.* 2(10): 819–829.

Vogel, T., Brechat, P. H, Leprêtre, P. M., Kaltenbach, G., Berthel, M., Lonsdorfer, J. 2009. "Health benefits of physical activity in older patients: a review." *International Journal of Clinical Practice* (63)2: 303–20.

Babraj, J. A., Vollaard, N. B. J., Keast, C., Gruppy, F., Cottrell, G. & Timmons, J. A. 2009. "Extremely short duration high intensity interval training substantially improves insulin action in young healthy males." *BMC Endocrine Disorders* 9 (3).

Walsh, N.P et al. 2011. "Position statement part one: immune function and exercise." *Exercise Immunology Review* 17 pp.6–63.

Michael Gleeson. 2007. "Immune function in sport and exercise." *J Appl Physiol* 103: 693–699.

Gordon, L. Klein. 2014. "Insulin and bone: Recent developments." *World J Diabetes* 5(1): 14–16.

Asghar, L. George, and M. F. Lokhandwala. 2007. "Exercise decreases oxidative stress and inflammation M. and restores renal dopamine D1 receptor function in old rats." *American Journal of Physiology Renal Physiology* (293)3: F914–F919.

Ross, A., Thomas, S. 2010. "The health benefits of yoga and exercise: a review of comparison studies." *J Altern Complement Med.* (Jan); 16(1): 3–12. Review.

Baker, L. D., Frank, L. L., Foster-Schubert, K., et al. 2010. "Effects of aerobic exercise on mild cognitive impairment: a controlled trial." *Arch Neurol.* 67(1): 71–79.

Gjevestad, G. O., Holven, K. B., Ulven, S. M. 2015. "Effects of exercise on gene expression of inflammatory markers in human peripheral blood cells: a systematic review." *Curr. Cardiovasc. Risk Rep* 9(7):34.

Erickson, K. I., Voss, M. W., Prakash, R. S., Basak, C., Szabo, A., Chaddock, L., Kim, J. S., Heo, S., Alves, H., White, S. M., Wojcicki, T. R., Mailey, E., Vieira, V. J., Martin, S. A., Pence, B. D., Woods, J. A., McAuley, E., Kramer, A. F., et al. 2011. "Exercise training increases size of hippocampus and improves memory." *Proc Natl Acad Sci* U S A108(7): 3017–22.

Shiroma, E. J., Sesso, H. D., Moorthy, M. V., Buring, J. E., Lee, I. M. 2014. "Do moderate-intensity and vigorous-intensity physical activities reduce mortality rates to the same extent?" *J Am Heart Assoc.* 3: e000984.

Tjonna, A. E., Leinan, I. M., Bartnes, A. T., Jenssen, B. M., Gibala, M. J., Winett, R. A., Wisloff, U. 2013. "Low and high-volume of intensive endurance training significantly improves maximal oxygen uptake after 10 weeks of training in healthy men." *PLoS One*. 8:1–7.

Paoli. A., Pacelli, Q. F., Moro, T., et al. 2013. "Effects of high-intensity circuit training, low-intensity circuit training and endurance training on blood pressure and lipoproteins in middle-aged overweight men." *Lipids Health Dis*. 12:131.

Wang, B. W. E., Ramey, D. R., Schettler, J. D., Hubert, H. B., Fries, J. F. 2002. "Postponed Development of Disability in Elderly Runners: A 13-Year Longitudinal Study." *Arch Intern Med*. 162(20): 2285–2294.

Ruangthai, R., Phoemsapthawee, J. 2019. "Combined exercise training improves blood pressure and antioxidant capacity in elderly individuals with hypertension." *Journal of Exercise Science & Fitness* 17; 2 67–76.

Booth, F. W., Chakravarthy, M. V., Spangenburg, E. E. 2002. "Exercise and gene expression: physiological regulation of the human genome through physical activity." *J Physiol*. (Sep 1); 543(Pt 2): 399–411. Review.

https://well.blogs.nytimes.com › 2014/12/17 › how-exercise-changes-our DNA-…

Kohl, H. W., Craig, C. L., Lambert, E. V., Inoue, S., Alkandari, J. R., Leetongin, G., Kahlmeier, S.; Lancet Physical Activity Series Working Group. 2012. "The pandemic of physical inactivity: global action for public health." *Lancet* 380(9838): 294–305.

Campbell, J. P., Turner, J. E. 2018. "Debunking the Myth of Exercise-Induced Immune Suppression: Redefining the Impact of Exercise on Immunological Health Across the Lifespan." *Front Immun*.

Messier, S. P., Gutekunst, D. J., Davis, C., DeVita, P. 2005. "Weight loss reduces knee-joint loads in overweight and obese older adults with knee osteoarthritis." *Arthritis Rheum*. (Jul); 52(7): 2026–32.

https://www.nhlbi.nih.gov ›› Healthy Weight Tools › BMI Calculator.

Powell, K. E., Blair, S. N. "The public health burdens of sedentary living habits: theoretical but realistic estimates." *Med Sci Sports Exerc.* 26 (1994): 851–856.

US National Library of Medicine. National Institutes of Health Collection Development Manual. Complementary and Alternative Medicine. 8 October 2003. Online Version. Retrieved 31 July 2015.

Min Lee, I., Shiroma, E. J., Blair, Katzmarzyk, P. T. "Effect of physical inactivity on major non-communicable diseases worldwide: an analysis of burden of disease and life expectancy." *Lancet* (2012) 380(9838): 219–229.

Oberg, E. 2007. "Physical Activity Prescription: Our best Medicine." *Int Med* 6:5:18–19.

Knowler, W. C., Barrett-Connor, E., Fowler, S. E., Hamman, R. F., Lachin, J. M., Walker, E. A., Nathan, D. M.; Diabetes Prevention Program Research Group. 2002. "Reduction in the incidence of type 2 diabetes with lifestyle intervention or metformin." *N. Engl. J. Med.* 346(6): 393–403.

Office of the Surgeon General (US); Office of Disease Prevention and Health Promotion (US); Centers for Disease Control and Prevention (US); National Institutes of Health (US). The Surgeon General's Call to Action to Prevent and Decrease Overweight and Obesity. Rockville (MD): Office of the Surgeon General (US). 2001. Available from: https://www.ncbi.nlm.nih.gov/books/NBK44206/.

Esmond-White, Miranda. *Aging Backwards*. Harper-Collins Books, 2014.

Lindstedt, S. L. LaStayo, P.C.; Reich, T.E. 2001. "When Active Muscles Lengthen: Properties and Consequences of Eccentric Contractions." *News Physiol. Sci. 16: 260.*

Zepetzauer, M.; Drexel, H.; Vonbank, A.; Rein, P.; Aczel, S.; Saely, C. H. 2013. "Eccentric endurance exercise economically improves metabolic and inflammatory risk factors." *Eur. J. Prev. Cardiol. 20 (4): 577–84.*

Chapter 5

Sroufe, L. A. 2001. "From infant attachment to promotion of adolescent autonomy: Prospective, longitudinal data on the role of parents in development." In J. G. Borkowski, S. L. Ramey & M. Bristol-Power (Eds.), *Parenting and the Child's World: Influences on Academic, Intellectual, and Social-emotional Development.* Psychology Press.

Masten, A. S. 2011. "Resilience in children threatened by extreme adversity: frameworks for research, practice, and translational synergy." *Development and Psychopathology* 23(2): 493–506.

Diamond, Marian C. 2001. "Response of the Brain to Enrichment." *Anais da Academia Brasileira de Ciencias* (73)2.

Jones, E. G. 1986. "Neurotransmitters in the cerebral cortex." *J. Neurosurg.* 65(2):135–53. Abstract.

Perth, C. *Molecules of Emotion: The Science Behind Mind-Body Medicine.* Schribner, 2003.

Carhart-Harris, R. L. and Nutt, D. J. 2017. "Serotonin and brain function: a tale of two receptors." *J Psychopharmacol.* 31(9): 1091–1120.

Lazar, V., Ditu, L. M., Pircalabioru, G. G., et al. 2018. "Aspects of Gut Microbiota and Immune System Interactions in Infectious Diseases, Immunopathology, and Cancer." *Front Immunol.* 9(2018): 1830.

Clapp, M., Aurora, N., Herrera, L., Bhatia, M., Wilen, E., Wakefield, S. 2017. "Gut microbiota's effect on mental health: The gut-brain axis." *Clin. Pract.* 7(4):987.

Cani, P. D., Bibiloni, R., Knauf, C., Waget, A., Neyrinck, A. M., Delzenne, N. M., Burcelin, R. 2008. "Changes in gut microbiota control metabolic endotoxemia-induced inflammation in high-fat diet-induced obesity and diabetes in mice." *Diabetes.* 57(6): 1470–81.

Martin, C. R., Osadchiy, V., Kalani, A., and Mayer, E. A. 2018. "The Brain-Gut-Microbiome Axis (2018)." *Cell Mol Gastroenterol Hepatol.* 6(2): 133–148.

David Kohn. "When Gut Bacteria Change Brain Function." Article, *The Atalantic Visit Site* (June 24, 2015).

Mishra, A., Singh, S. and Shukla, S. 2018. "Physiological and Functional Basis of Dopamine Receptors and Their Role in Neurogenesis: Possible Implication for Parkinson's disease." *J Exp Neurosci.* 2018; 12: 1179069518779829.

"Leveraging the Psychology of the Salesperson: A Conversation with Psychologist and Anthropologist G. Clotaire Rapaille." *Sales & Marketing Magazine.* Article Diane L. Couta.

Naumann, R. K., Ondracek, J. M., Reiter, S., Shein-Idelson, M., Tosches, M. A., Yamawaki, T. M., Laurent, G. 2002. "The reptilian brain." *Curr. Biol.* 25(8): R317–R321.

Bargh, J. A., and Morsella, E. 2008. "The Unconscious Mind." *Perspect Psychol Sci.* Jan; 3(1): 73–79.

Avena, N. M., Rada, P., et al. 2009. "Sugar and Fat Binging Have Notable Differences in Addictive Behaviour." *J Nutr.* 39(3): 623–28.

Opioid Crisis. Official web site of the U.S. Health Resources. https://www.hrsa.gov/opioids

Michael O. Schroeder. Death By Prescription. Staff Writer, *US News and World Report*, Sept. 27, 2016.

"Pain Management and the Opioid Epidemic." NCBI. https://www.ncbi.nlm.nih.gov/books/NBK458661.

Knuppel, A., Shipley, M., Llewellyn, C. H., Brunner, E. J. 2017. "Sugar intake from sweet food and beverages, common mental disorder and depression: prospective findings from the Whitehall II study." Scientific Reports (7):6287.

Buric, I., Farias, M., Jong, J., Mee, C., Brazil, I. A. 2017. "What Is the Molecular Signature of Mind-Body Interventions? A Systematic Review of Gene Expression Changes Induced by Meditation and Related Practices." *Front Immunol.* 8:670. Review.

Renoir, T., Hasebe, K., Gray, L. 2013. "Mind and body: how the health of the body impacts on neuropsychiatry." *Front Pharmacol.* 4:158.

Schneiderman, N., Ironson, G., Siegel, S. D. 2005. "Psychological, Behavioral and Biological Determinants." *Annu. Rev. Clin. Psychol.* 1: 607–628.

Goyal, M. 2014. "Meditation programs for psychological stress and well-being: a systematic review and meta-analysis." *JAMA Intern Med.* 174(7): 1193–4.

C. Hayes, S., Mathews, A., Perman, G. and Hirsch, C. R. "The power of positive thinking: Pathological worry is reduced by thought replacement in Generalized Anxiety Disorder." *Behav. Res. Ther.* (2016 Mar); 78: 13–18.

de la Fuente-Fernández, R., Stoessl, A. J. 2004. "The biochemical bases of the placebo effect." Abstract. *Sci. Eng. Ethics.* 10(1): 143–50.

Colloca, L. "Preface: The Fascinating Mechanisms and Implications of the Placebo Effect." *Int Rev Neurobiol.* (2018) 138: xv–xx.

Voudouris, N. J., Peck, C. L., Coleman, G. 1989. "Conditioned response models of placebo phenomena: further support." *Pain* 38 (1): 109–16.

Wager, T. D., Atlas, L. Y. 2015. "The neuroscience of placebo effects: connecting context, learning and health." *Nature Reviews Neuroscience* (16): 403–418.

Atasoy, O. "Your Thought Can Release Abilities Beyond Normal Limits." Essay, *Scientific American* (Aug 13, 2013).

Crum, Alia J., and Ellen J. Langer. 2007. "Mind-set matters: Exercise and the placebo effect." *Psychological Science* 18, no. 2: 165–171.

Williams, L. E., Bargh, J. A. 2008. "Experiencing Physical Warmth Promotes Interpersonal Warmth." *Science* 322(5901): 606–607.

Diederich, N. J., Goetz, C. G. August 2008. "The placebo treatments in neurosciences: New insights from clinical and neuroimaging studies." *Neurology.* 71(9): 677–84.

Moseley, J. B., O'Malley, K., Petersen, N. J., et al. "A controlled trial of arthroscopic surgery for osteoarthritis of the knee." *N Engl J Med.* (2002 Jul 11); 347(2): 81–8.

McEwen, B. S. 2012. "Brain on stress: how the social environment gets under the skin." *Proc Natl Acad Sci* U S A *109*(2): 17180–17185.

Poitras, V. J., Pyke, K. E. 2013. "The impact of acute mental stress on vascular endothelial function: evidence, mechanisms and importance." *Int. J. Psychophysiol.* 88: 124–135.

Evans, W. & Rosenberg, I. *10 Biomarkers of Ageing.* Simon & Schuster, 1991.

Moore, R. A., Wiffen P. J., Derry, S., Maguire, T., Roy, Y. M., Tyrrell, L. 2015. "Non-prescription (OTC) oral analgesics for acute pain—an overview of Cochrane reviews." *Cochrane Database Syst Rev.* (11): CD010794. Review.

Derecki, N. C., Cardani, A. N., Yang, C. H., Quinnies, K. M., Crihfield, A., Lynch, K. R., Kipnis. J. 2010. "Regulation of learning and memory by meningeal immunity: a key role for IL-4." *J Exp Med.* 207(5): 1067–80.

Slavich, G. M., Irwin, M. R. 2014. "From stress to inflammation and major depressive disorder: a social signal transduction theory of depression." *Psychol Bull* 140(3): 774–815. doi:10.1037/a0035302.

Staples, J. K. "The Science of Mantra." Science for the Yoga Therapist

C. R. Karnick. 1983. "Effects of Mantras on Humans and Plants." *Anc Sci Life.* 2(3): 141–147.

Ashley-Farrand, G. *Healing Mantras: Using Sound Affirmations for Personal Power, Creativity, and Healing.* Gill and Macmillan, 2000.

Bai S, Guo W, Feng Y, et al. Efficacy and safety of anti-inflammatory agents for the treatment of major depressive disorder: a systematic review and meta-analysis of randomised controlled trials. *J Neurol Neurosurg Psychiatry.* 2020;91(1):21-32.

Common Traits of School Shooters The Heritage Foundation *www.heritage.org › education › commentary*

Everson-Rose, S., Nicholas, S. Roetker, N. S., Lutsey, P. L., Kershaw, K., Longstreth, W. K., Jr, R. L, Diez Roux, A. V, and Alonso, A. 2014. "Chronic Stress, Depressive Symptoms, Anger, Hostility and Risk of Stroke and Transient Ischemic Attack in the MESA Study Stroke." 45(8): 2318–2323.

Salleh, M. R. 2008. "Life event, Stress and Illness." *Malays J Med Sci* 15(4): 9–18.

Mary Carol R. Hunter et al., "Urban Nature Experiences Reduce Stress in the Context of Daily Life Based on Salivary Biomarkers," *Frontiers in Psychology*, April 4, 2019.

Eva Selhub. "Nutritional Psychiatry: Your brain on food." Article. *Harvard Health Blog*.

Derbyshire, D. 2012. "Loneliness is a killer: It's as bad for your health as alcoholism, smoking and over-eating, say scientists." Health mail online, updated 9:36 GMT. (2010. Jul 28). *Lancet Articles* 380(9838): 219–229.

Holt-Lunstad, J., Smith, T. B., Baker, M., Harris, T., Stephenson. 2015. "Perspect Psychol Sci. Loneliness and Social Isolation as Risk Factors for Mortality: A Meta-Analytic Review." 10(2) 227–237.

Chapter 6

Littman, R. J. 2009. "The plague of Athens: epidemiology and paleopathology." *Sinai J Med*. O6(5): 456–67.

Sabbatani, S., Fiorino, S. 2009. "The Antonine Plague and the decline of the Roman Empire." *Infez. Med.* 17(4):261–75.

Ancient History Encyclopedia. Mark Cartwright. Essay (20 June 2018): Black Death.

Rogers, D. J., Wilson, A. J., Hay, S. I., Graham, A. J. "The global distribution of yellow fever and dengue."

Enard D, Cai L, Gwennap C, Petrov DA. Viruses are a dominant driver of protein adaptation in mammals. *Elife*. 2016;5:e12469. Published 2016 May 17. doi:10.7554/eLife.12469

Content source: *CDC Global Health*. "Division of Parasitic Diseases and Malaria" (November 14, 2018).

Chen, L. H., Blair. B. M. 2015. "Infectious Risks of Traveling Abroad." *Microbiol Spectr*. (Aug); 3(4). Review.

World Health Organization. *Infectious Diseases. https://www.who.int/ whr/1996/media_centre/press_release/en/*

Advances in Parasitology. Volume 62 (2006). Pages 181–220. "The Global Distribution of Yellow Fever and Dengue."

Sven Hernberg, MD, MPH. "Lead Poisoning in a Historical Perspective." *American Journal of Industrial Med* (2000) 38:244± 254.

WHO: Climate change and human health—risks and responses. Summary.

Zeng, J., Suh, S. 2019. "Strategies to reduce the global carbon footprint of plastics." *Nature Climate Change* 9, 374–378.

Hoegh-Guldberg, O. D.; Jacob, M.; Taylor, M.; S., Bindi; Brown, I. 2018. "The Impact of Global Warming of 1.5°C." *In Press.*

Hoegh-Guldberg, O. 1999. "Coral bleaching, climate change and the future of the world's coral reefs." *Marine and Freshwater Research* 50: 839–866.

IPCC 2018. "Global Warming of 1.5°C, an IPCC special report on the impacts of global warming of 1.5°C above pre-industrial levels and related global greenhouse gas emission pathways, in the context of strengthening the global response to the threat of climate

Drug resistance: Does antibiotic use in animals affect human health?" Published Friday 9 November 2018 by Ana Sandoiu in Medical News Today.

Derek R. MacFadden, Sarah F. McGough, David Fisman, Mauricio Santillana and John S. Brownstein. "H Antibiotic resistance increases with local temperature." *Letter Nature Climate Change.* https://doi.org/10.1038/s41558-018-0161-6.

"Haiti: Cholera figures (as of 31 January 2019)." Infographic from UN Office for the Coordination of Humanitarian Affairs. Published 31 Jan 2019.

Chagnon, M., Kreutzweiser, D., Mitchell, E. A., Morrissey, C. A., Noome, D. A., Van der Sluijs, J. P. 2015. "Risks of large-scale use of systemic insecticides to ecosystem functioning and services." *Environ. Sci. Pollut. Res. Int.* (Jan); 22(1): 119–34.

Broughton, E. "The Bhopal disaster and its aftermath: a review." *Environ Health* (2005 May 10); 4(1):6.

https://www.publichealth.va.gov › exposures › agent orange › conditions.

https://labblog.uofmhealth.org/…/study-examines-blood-lead-levels-of-flint-children.

NBC (14 April 2018): "More evidence firefighters risk cancer from 9/11 exposure. Male first responders may risk multiple myeloma, prostate, thyroid cancer."

Harari, Y. N. *Sapiens: A Brief History of Humankind.* Harper, 2015.

CDC Third National Climate Assessment's Health Chapter. Climate Effects on Health

Bill Davenhall. 2012. "Geomedicine." Geography and Personal Health Esri.

Berke, Ethan M. *2010*. "Geographic Information Systems (GIS): Recognizing the Importance of Place in Primary Care Research and Practice." *The Journal of the American Board of Family Medicine (January* 23); (1) 9–12.

WHO report on Drinking Water. June 14, 2019.

Elizabeth Grossman. "Radioactivity in the Ocean: Diluted, But Far from Harmless." *Yale environment 360* (April 7, 2011).

IAEA: Inventory of Radioactive waste disposal at sea. Aug 1999.

Goodman, J., Conway, C. "Poor Health: When Poverty Becomes Disease." *Patient Care.* January 6, 2016. Article.

"Environmental Studies Faculty Publications Racial Inequality in the Distribution of Hazardous Waste: A National Level Reassessment." Paul Mohai Follow Robin Saha, University of Montana-Missoula 2007.

Luber, G., Prudent, N. 2009. "Climate Change and Human Health." *Trans. Am. Clin. Climatol. Assoc.* 120: 113–11.

The Impacts of Climate Change on Human Health in the United States. https://health2016.globalchange.gov/. A Scientific Assessment.

US call to action on climate, health and equity: A policy Action 2019. the *AMA.*

https://www.ama-assn.org › delivering-care › public-health › why-physicias see climate as a health emergency.

Van Renssen, S. 2019. "Looking past the horizon of 2100." *Nature Climate Change* 9: 349–351. Millenium Alliance for Humanity and the Biosphere (MAHEB) mahb.stanford.edu

Overpopulation and the Collapse of Civilization Ehrlich, Paul R. November 5, 2013

"Harvard Health Publishing: Hugs heartfelt in more ways than one." Published March 2014.

How We Know Today's Climate Change Is Not Natural. https://blogs.ei.columbia.edu › 2017/04/04.

Wilkinson, R. and Pickett, K. (2010) *The Spirit Level: Why Equality Is Better For Everyone*. London: Penguin Books

Chapter 7

Marketos, S. G. 1997. "The parallels between Asclepian and Hippocratic medicine on the island of Kos." *Am J Nephrol.*; 17(3–4): 205–8. Abstract.

Kleisiaris, C. F., Sfakianakis, C., Papathanasiou, I. V. 2014. "Health care practices in ancient Greece: The Hippocratic ideal." *J Med Ethics Hist Med.* 2014; 7:6.

Katsambas, A., Marketos, S. G. 2007. "Hippocratic messages for modern medicine (the vindication of Hippocrates)." *J Eur Acad Dermatol Venereol.* (6): 859–61. Abstract.

*Bak RO, Gomez-Ospina N, Porteus MH (2018). "Gene Editing on Center Stage". Trends in Genetics. **34** (8): 600–611.*

ABOUT THE AUTHOR

An innovative and holistic thinker, Dr. Elvebakk came to medicine with the long-held belief that illnesses are explainable in terms of our environment and behavior. Her road to this book was a long one, starting in earnest when she saw the effect of nutrition on overweight and metabolically ill patients.

Dr. Elvebakk is a former primary-care physician who spent most of her career working with weight and related illnesses. In 2008 she wrote her first book, *The Food Tree*, debunking fads and myths and raising nutrition to the scientific level. She is gratified that the views expressed in the book are passing the test of time.

She then started looking for other triggers of illness. This led to a rich network of connections between the environment and inflammation and to the discovery of the role of modern physics, including quantum, in explaining the interactions between the body and the environment. It ultimately led to the writing of this book.

After receiving her medical degree from University of Oslo, Norway, Dr. Elvebakk performed post-graduate training in Norway and in the United States, including an internship in internal medicine at UC Davis California. She was a long-standing member of the American Society of Bariatric Physicians, The American Academy of Family Care Physicians, and the AMA.

Dr. Elvebakk was born in Scandinavia and is a proponent of physical fitness and the outdoors. She is a consummate health advocate. As a columnist and expert commentator, she has written and lectured on weight and nutrition in the United States and in Europe. She spends her time writing and talking on nutrition and illness.

This inspiring book holds the key to changing our health at the most fundamental level. The simple treatment of a complicated topic makes it a must-read for everyone. She hopes the information will make us powerful advocates for ourselves and the planet.

www.ingramcontent.com/pod-product-compliance
Lightning Source LLC
Chambersburg PA
CBHW070705250726
48662CB00001B/272